HELLO KIDS COOKBOOK

Fun and Easy Recipes for Little Chefs

By

Lucia Johnson-Flores

Hello Kids Cookbook

By

Lucia Johnson-Flores

Copyright © 2024

Happy Tales, LLC

www.happytales.biz

PO Box 390428

Edina, MN 55439

ISBN: 978-1-965256-12-1 (Paperback)

ISBN: 978-1-965256-13-8 (Hardcover)

ISBN: 978-1-965256-14-5 (Digital Version)

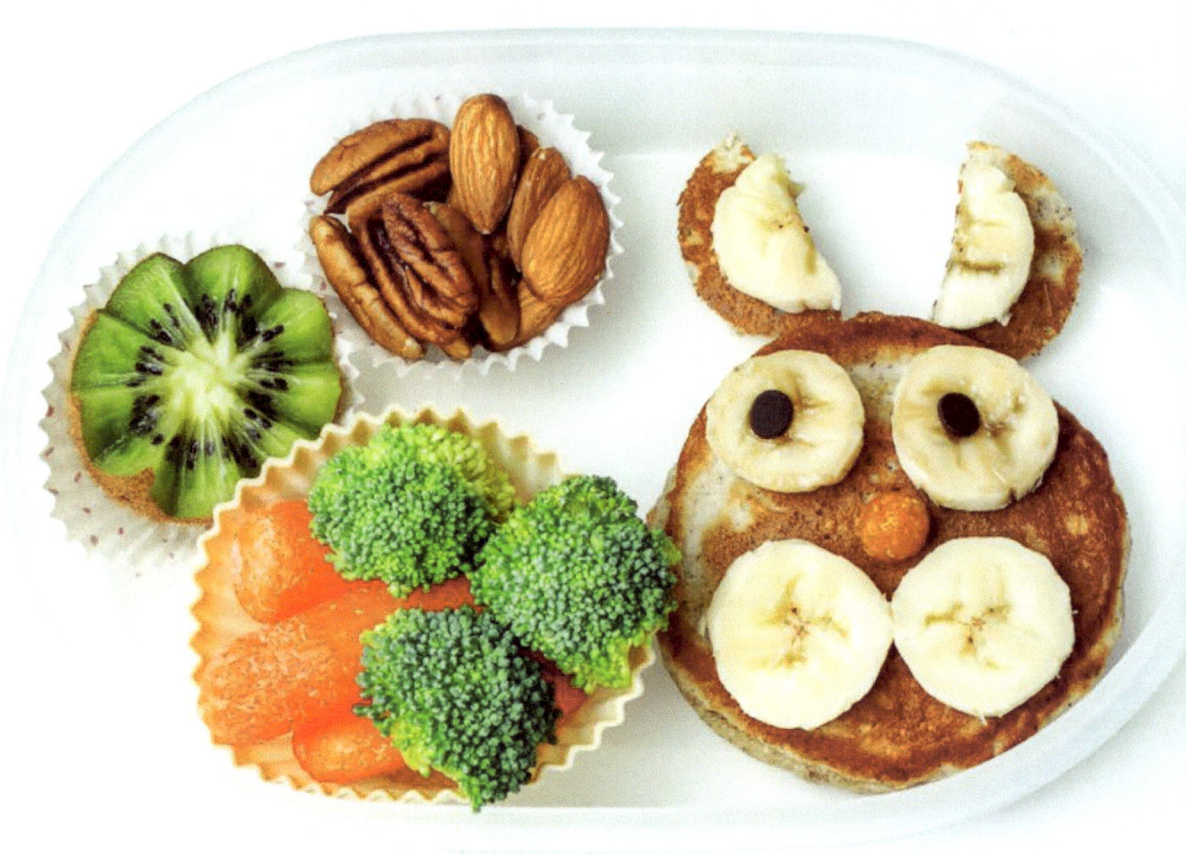

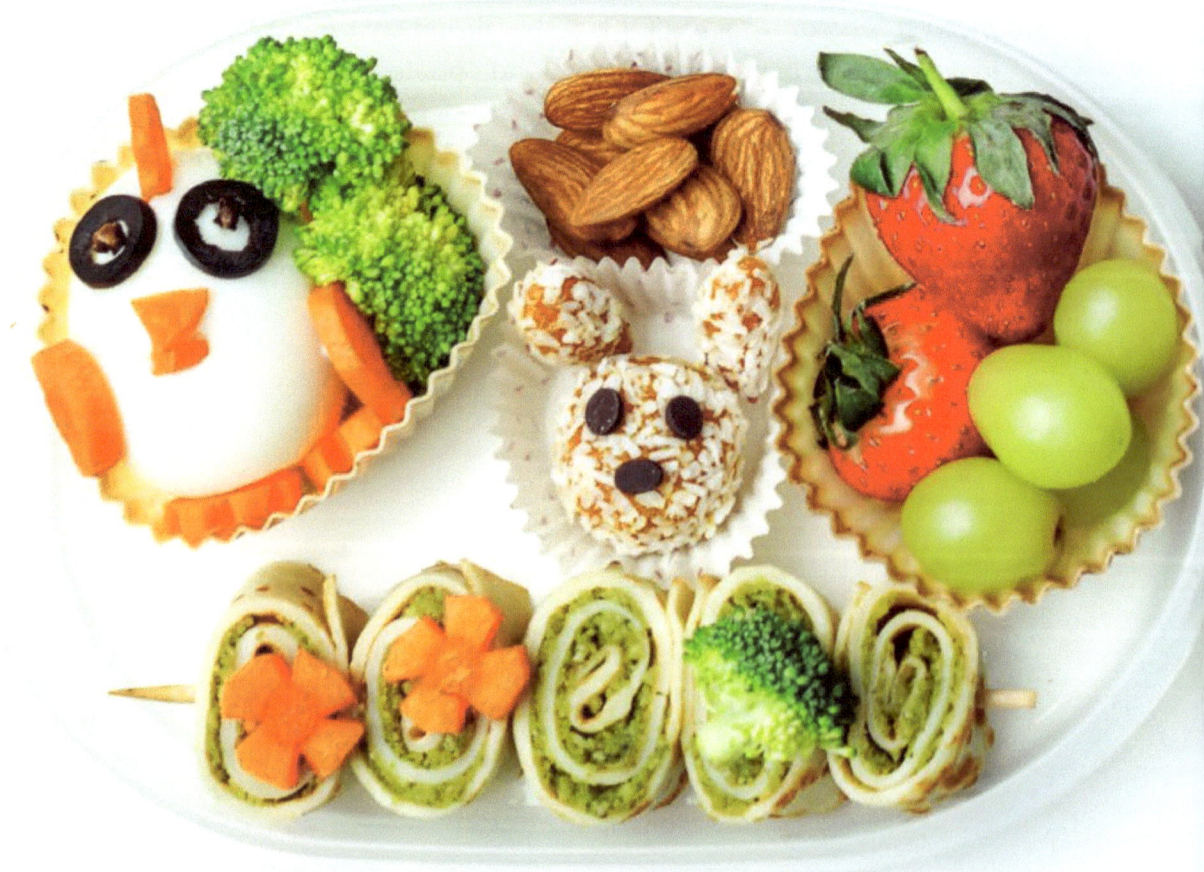

INTRODUCTION

Welcome to the "Hello Kids Cookbook," the ultimate kitchen companion for budding chefs! Packed with 50 delightful and easy-to-follow recipes, this cookbook is designed to spark a love for cooking in children of all ages.

From breakfast treats and lunchbox delights to tasty snacks and delicious dinners, each recipe is crafted to be both fun and educational. But cooking isn't just about following recipes—it's about learning valuable skills too. "Hello Kids Cookbook" includes essential information on cooking measurements, kitchen tools, and safety precautions to ensure that young chefs can cook with confidence and care. Discover how to measure ingredients accurately,how to identify kitchen tools, and how to stay safe while cooking up a storm.

With colorful illustrations and simple instructions, this cookbook makes learning to cook a joyous adventure. Kids will love making their own creations and sharing them with family and friends. Plus, they'll gain a sense of accomplishment and independence as they master new skills.

"Hello Kids Cookbook" is more than just a collection of recipes—it's a gateway to a lifelong love of cooking. Join us on this culinary journey and inspire the young chefs in your life to create, explore, and enjoy the wonderful world of food.

So tie on your apron, wash your hands and say "Hello" to the fun and rewarding world of cooking!

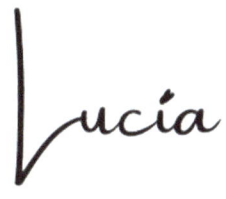

Contents

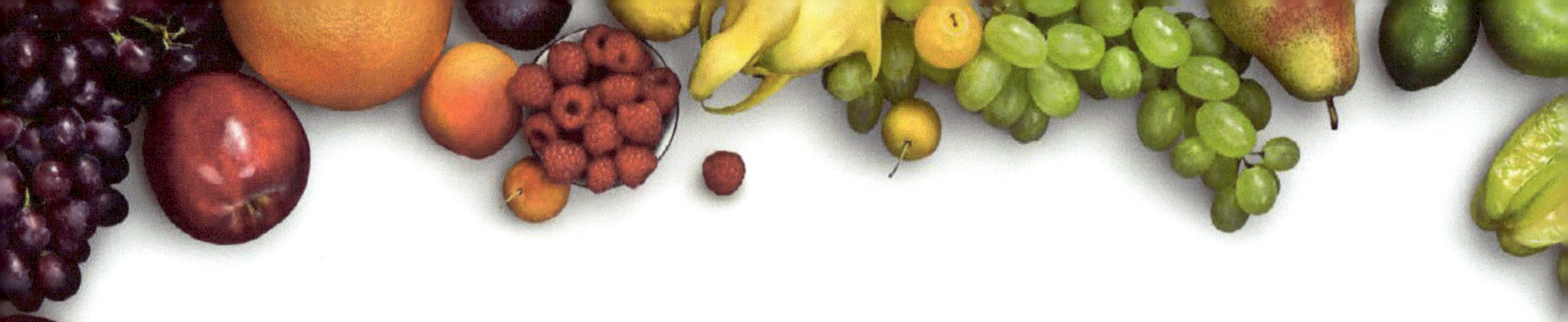

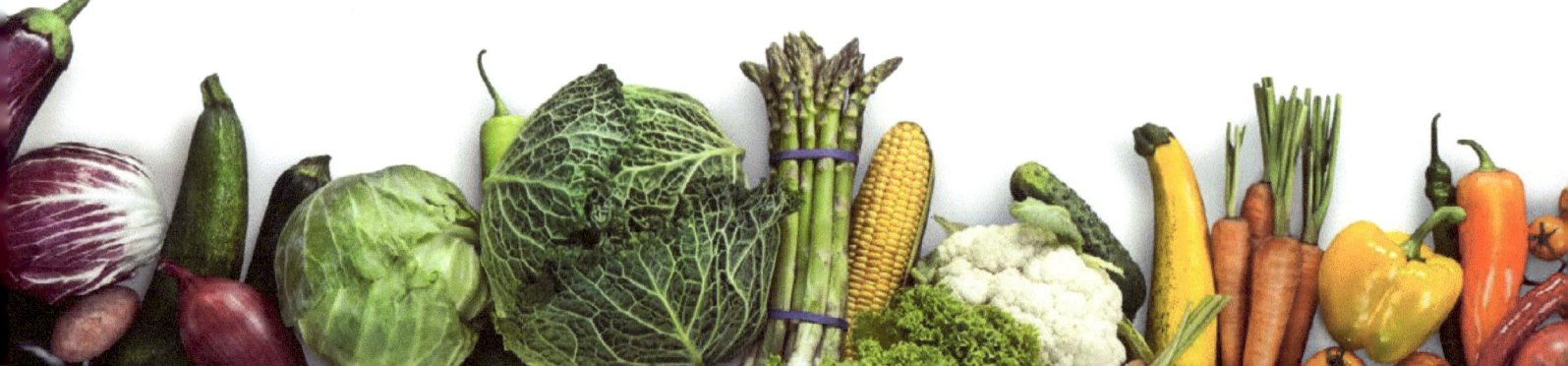

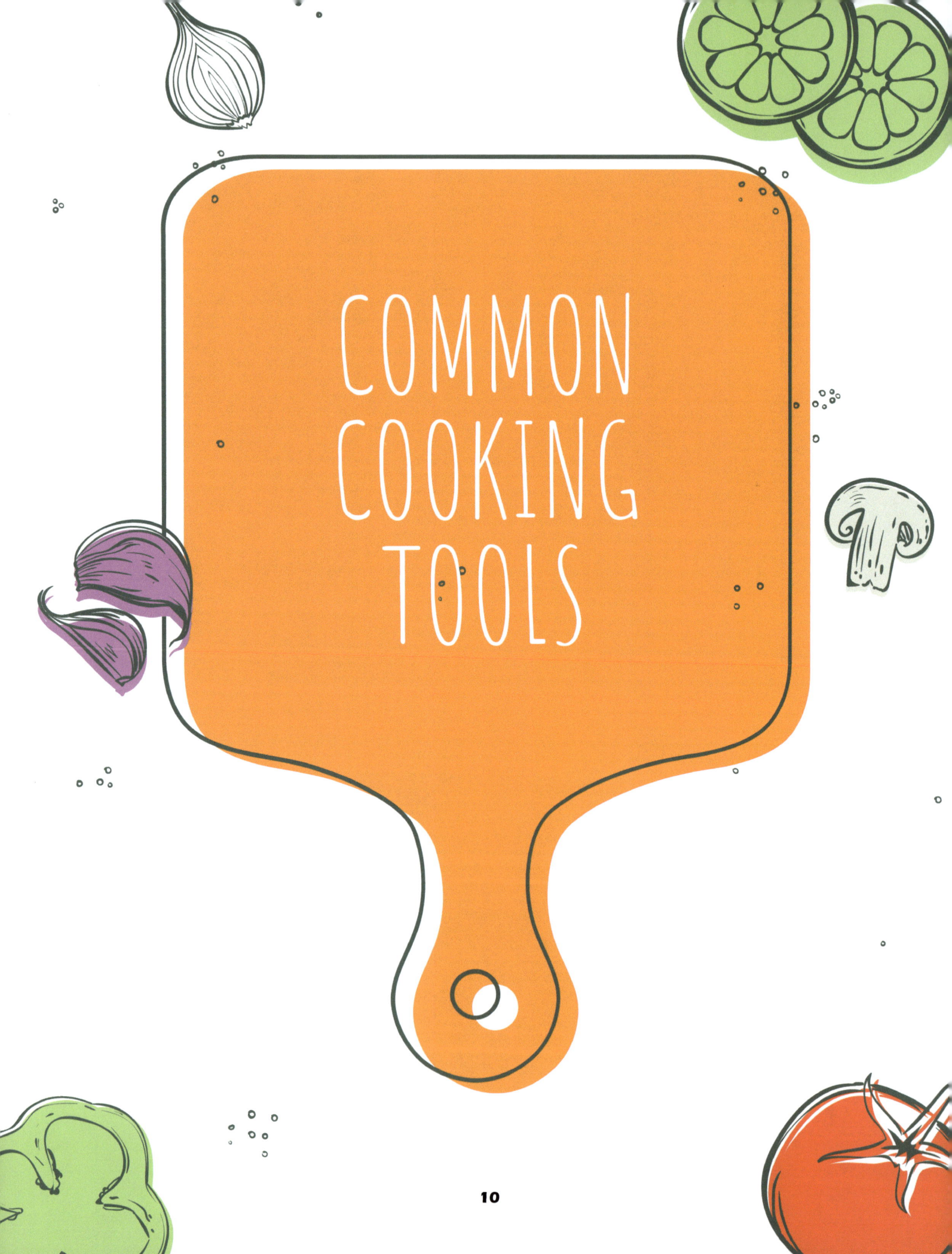

COMMON COOKING TOOLS

Common Kitchen Tools

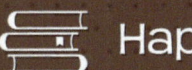 HappyTales

Baking sheets	Barbecue	Blender	Bottle opener	Bowls	Can opener	Cleaver
		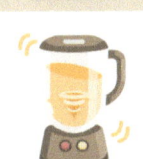	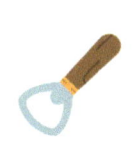	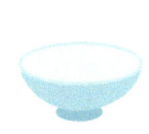	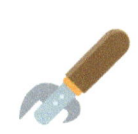	
Coffee cup	Coffee maker	Colander	Cooktop	Cutting board	Electric kettle	Electric whisk
	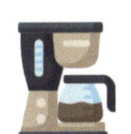	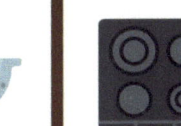	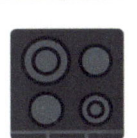	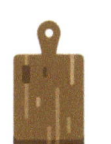	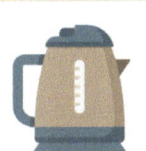	
Fork	Food containers	Frying pan	Gas bottle	Garlic press	Glass	Grater
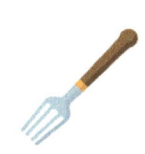	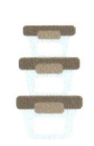	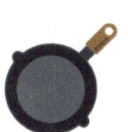	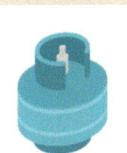	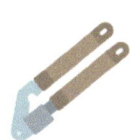	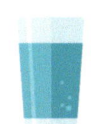	
Grill	Kettle	Knife	Ladle	Masher	Mortar	Mug
	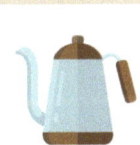	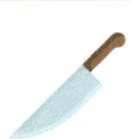	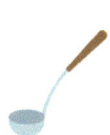	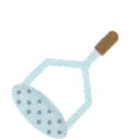	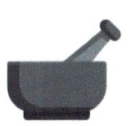	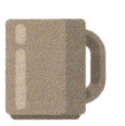
Oven	Oven mitt	Plate	Pitcher	Rolling pin	Salt shaker	Saucepan
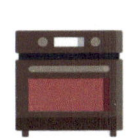				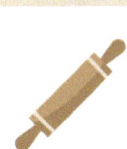	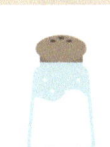	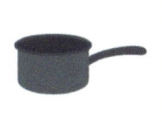
Sieve	Skimmer	Spoon	Spatula	Stock pot	Strainer	Teacup
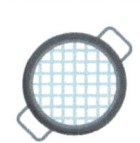	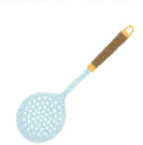	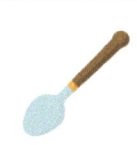		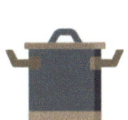	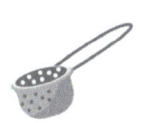	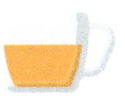
Teapot	Thermos	Tongs	Toaster	Tray	Vegetable peeler	Whisk
	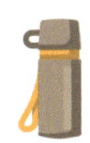	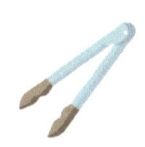	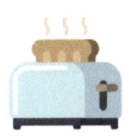	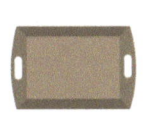	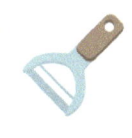	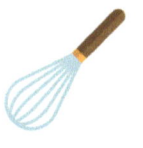

BASIC COOKING TERMS

Basic Cooking Terms

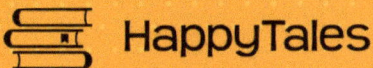 HappyTales

 Bake
To cook in an oven.

 Beat
To mix ingredients together using a fast, circular movement with a spoon, fork, whisk or mixer.

 Blanch
To briefly cook food in boiling water, then immediately plunge it into ice water to stop the cooking process.

 Blend
To mix ingredients together gently with a spoon, fork, or until combined.

 Boil
To heat a food so that the liquid gets hot enough for bubbles to rise and break the surface.

 Broil
To cook under direct heat.

 Brown
To cook over medium or high heat until surface of food browns or darkens.

 Caramelize
To melt sugar over medium heat in a skillet, stirring constantly, until it is a pale brown syrup.

 Chop
To cut into small pieces.

 Dice
To cut into small cubes.

 Drain
To remove all the liquid using a colander, strainer, or by pressing a plate against the food while tilting the container.

 Grate or Shred
To scrape food against the holes of a grater making thin pieces.

 Grease
To lightly coat with oil, butter, margarine, or non-stick spray so food does not stick when cooking or baking.

 Julienne
To cut vegetables into thin, lengthwise strips.

 Knead
To press, fold and stretch dough until it is smooth and uniform, usually done by pressing with the heels of the hands.

 Marinate
To soak food in a liquid to tenderize or add flavor to it (the liquid is called a "marinade").

 Mash
To squash food with a fork, spoon, or masher.

 Mince
To cut into very small pieces, smaller than chopped or diced pieces.

 Mix
To stir ingredients together with a spoon, fork, or electric mixer until well combined.

 Preheat
To turn oven on ahead of time so that it is at the desired temperature when needed (usually takes about 5 to 10 minutes).

 Sauté
To cook quickly in a little oil, butter, or margarine.

 Simmer
To cook in liquid over low heat (low boil) so that bubbles just begin to break the surface.

 Stew
To cook in a small amount of liquid. The water may boil or simmer, as indicated for the food that is to be cooked.

 Steam
To cook food over steam without putting the food directly in water (usually done with a steamer).

 Stir
To mix by using a circular motion - going around and around until the ingredients are blended together.

 Stir Fry
To quickly cook small pieces of food over high heat while constantly stirring the food until it is crisply tender (usually done with a wok).

 Stock
The liquid in which meat, poultry, fish, or vegetables have been cooked. Meat stock is used for soup.

 Toast
To brown by direct heat.

 Toss
To lightly mix ingredients with 2 forks or a fork and spoon.

 Whip
To beat rapidly to introduce air bubbles into the food whipped. Applied to cream, eggs, and gelatin dishes.

FOOD SAFETY

Keeping Food Safe

Here are some ways to prevent food contamination.

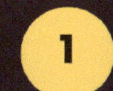 1 Keep it clean.

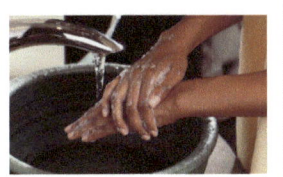 Wash your hands with soap and water before and after handling food.

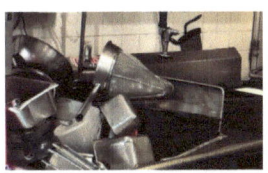 Wash kitchen utensils and keep surfaces clean

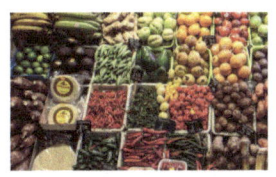 Wash fruits and vegetables in running water.

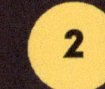 2 Avoid mix-ups.

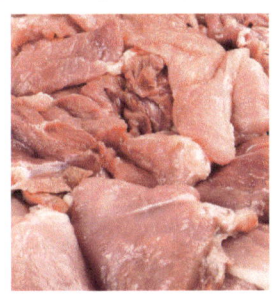 Separate raw meat, seafood and poultry from other food.

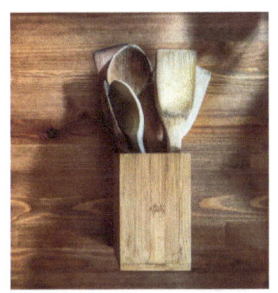 Use individual serving utensils.

3 Cook it well.

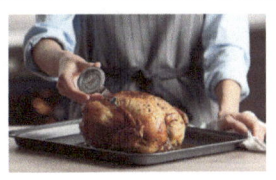 Cook food to the right temperature.

MINIMUM INTERNAL TEMPERATURE	Poultry: 165°F or 74°C
	Pork: 160°F or 71°C
	Beef: 145°F or 63°C

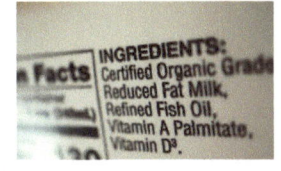 Follow package cooking instructions.

4 Keep it safe.

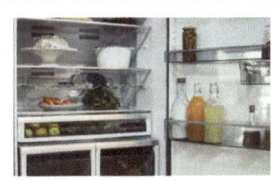 Place cooked food in separate containers.

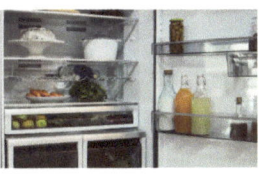 Refrigerate cooked food and leftovers.

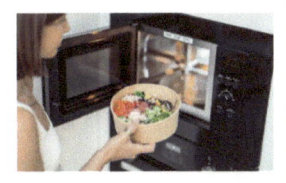 Reheat food before serving.

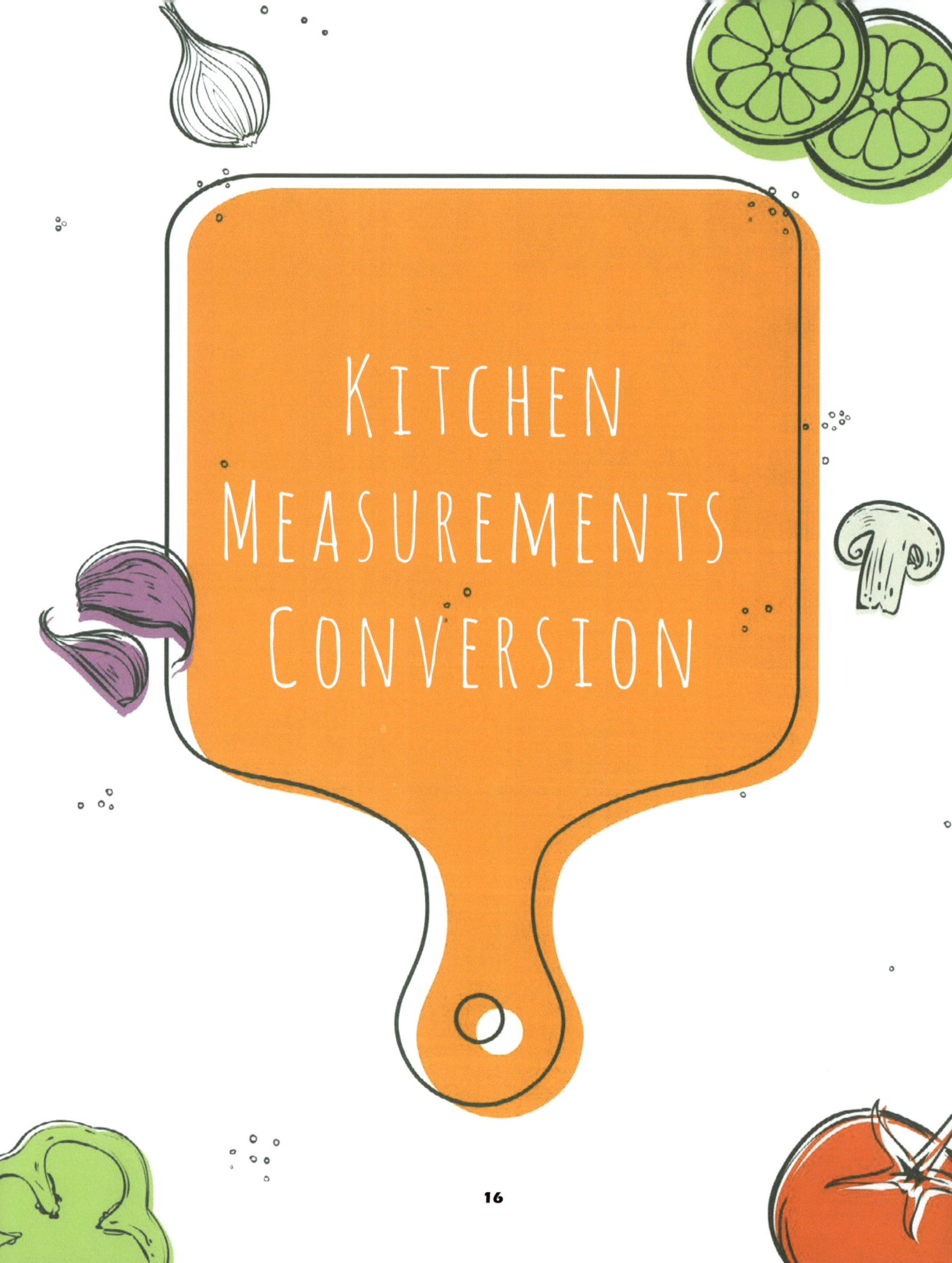

Kitchen Measurements Conversion

Kitchen Measurements and Conversions

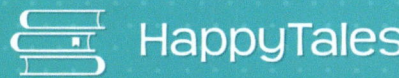 HappyTales

LIQUID VOLUMES

1 tsp = 5 mL

1 Tbsp = 15 mL

Dash = 1/8 tsp

Pinch = 1/16 tsp

DRY WEIGHTS

OZ	🥄	C	g	lb
1/2 OZ	1 tbsp	1/16 C	15 g	-
1 OZ	2 tbsp	1/8 C	28 g	-
2 OZ	4 tbsp	1/4 C	57 g	-
3 OZ	6 tbsp	1/3 C	85 g	-
4 OZ	8 tbsp	1/2 C	115 g	1/4 lb
8 OZ	16 tbsp	1 C	227 g	1/2 lb
12 OZ	24 tbsp	1 1/2 C	340 g	3/4 lb
16 OZ	32 tbsp	2 C	455 g	1 lb

EGG TIMER

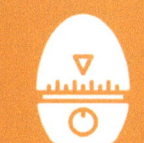

Soft 5 min.

Medium 7 min.

Hard 9 min.

oz	🥄	🥄	mL	C	pt	qt
1 oz	6 tsp	2 tsp	30 mL	1/8 C	-	-
2 oz	12 tsp	4 tsp	60 mL	1/4 C	-	-
2 2/3 oz	16 tsp	5 tsp	80 mL	1/3 C	-	-
4 oz	24 tsp	8 tsp	120 mL	1/2 C	-	-
5 1/3 oz	32 tsp	11 tsp	160 mL	2/3 C	-	-
6 oz	36 tsp	12 tsp	177 mL	3/4 C	-	-
8 oz	48 tsp	16 tsp	240 mL	1 C	1/2 pt	1/4 qt
16 oz	96 tsp	32 tsp	470 mL	2 C	1 pt	1/2 qt
32 oz	192 tsp	64 tsp	950 mL	4 C	2 pt	1 qt

OVEN TEMP

°F	°C	Gas Mark
500 -	- 260	🔥 10
475 -	- 240	🔥 9
450 -	- 230	🔥 8
425 -	- 220	🔥 7
400 -	- 200	🔥 6
375 -	- 190	🔥 5
350 -	- 180	🔥 4
325 -	- 170	🔥 3
300 -	- 150	🔥 2
275 -	- 140	🔥 1
250 -	- 120	🔥 1/2
225 -	- 110	🔥 1/4

For fan-forced ovens, reduce by

65°F | 20°C

LIQUID CONVERSIONS

1 GALLON
4 quarts
8 pints
16 cups
128 fl oz
3.8 liters

1 QUART
2 pints
4 cups
32 fl oz
946 mL

1 PINT
2 cups
16 fl oz
470 mL

1/4 CUP
4 tbsp 2 fl oz
12 tsp 60 mL

1 CUP
16 tbsp
8 fl oz
240 mL

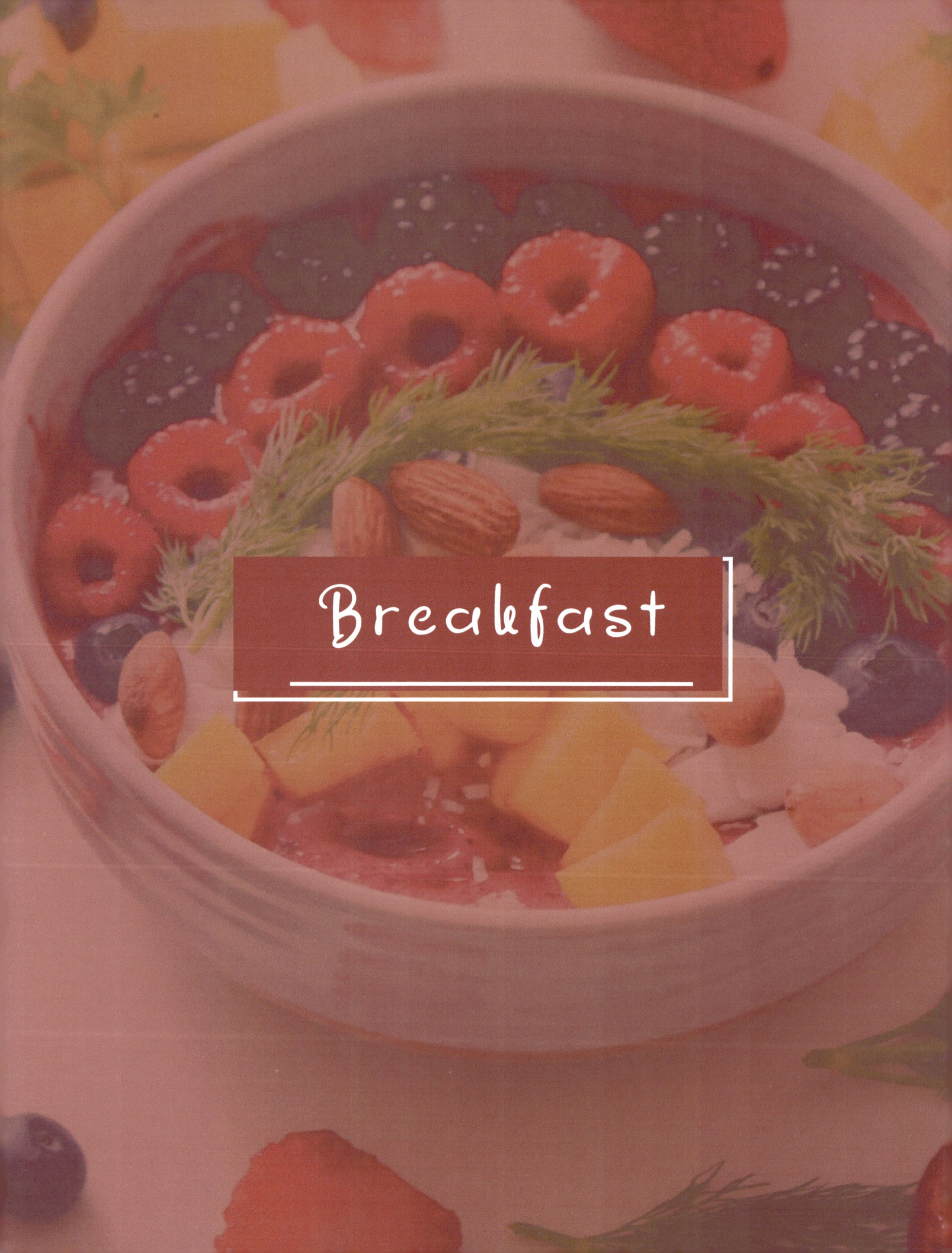

Breakfast

Chocolate Chip Pancakes

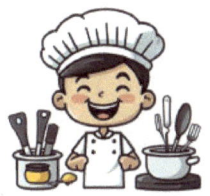

Ingredients

1 cup all-purpose flour
1 tablespoon sugar
1 teaspoon baking powder
1 cup milk
1 large egg
1/2 cup chocolate chips

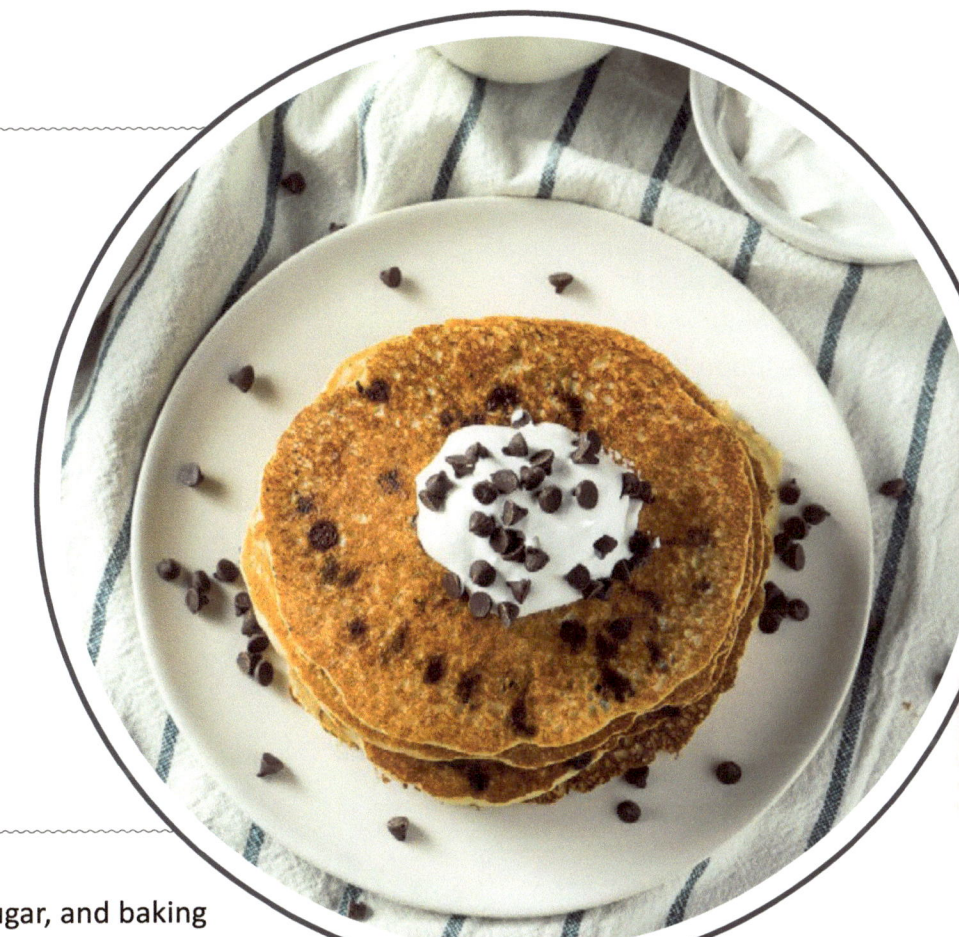

Instructions

1. In a deep-bottom bowl, mix the flour, sugar, and baking powder.
2. Add milk and egg to the dry elements mixture and whisk until smooth.
3. Gently fold in the chocolate chips.
4. Put the non-stick skillet over medium heat and pour 1/4 cup of batter for one pancake.
5. Cook until bubbles appear on the upper surface, then flip and cook until golden brown.

PREP TIME:
10 MINS

COOK TIME:
15 MINS

SERVING
2

Nutritional Values (per serving)

Calories: 250, Protein: 6g, Carbohydrates: 40g, Fat: 8g, Fiber: 2g

BERRY BLAST SMOOTHIE

INGREDIENTS

1 cup mixed berries (fresh or frozen)
1 banana
1 cup Greek yogurt
1/2 cup milk
1 tablespoon honey

INSTRUCTIONS

1. Place the mixed berries, banana, Greek yogurt, milk, and honey into a food blender.
2. Blend on high until smooth and creamy. Ladle the smoothie into two glasses.
3. Serve immediately and enjoy.

PREP TIME:
10 MINS

COOK TIME:
0 MINS

SERVING
2

NUTRITIONAL VALUES (PER SERVING)

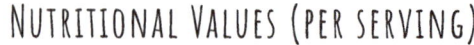

Calories: 180, Protein: 8g, Carbohydrates: 35g, Fat: 3g, Fiber: 5g

Peanut Butter Banana Toast

Ingredients

1 slice whole grain bread
2 tablespoons peanut butter
1 banana, sliced
1 teaspoon honey (optional)
A pinch of cinnamon (optional)

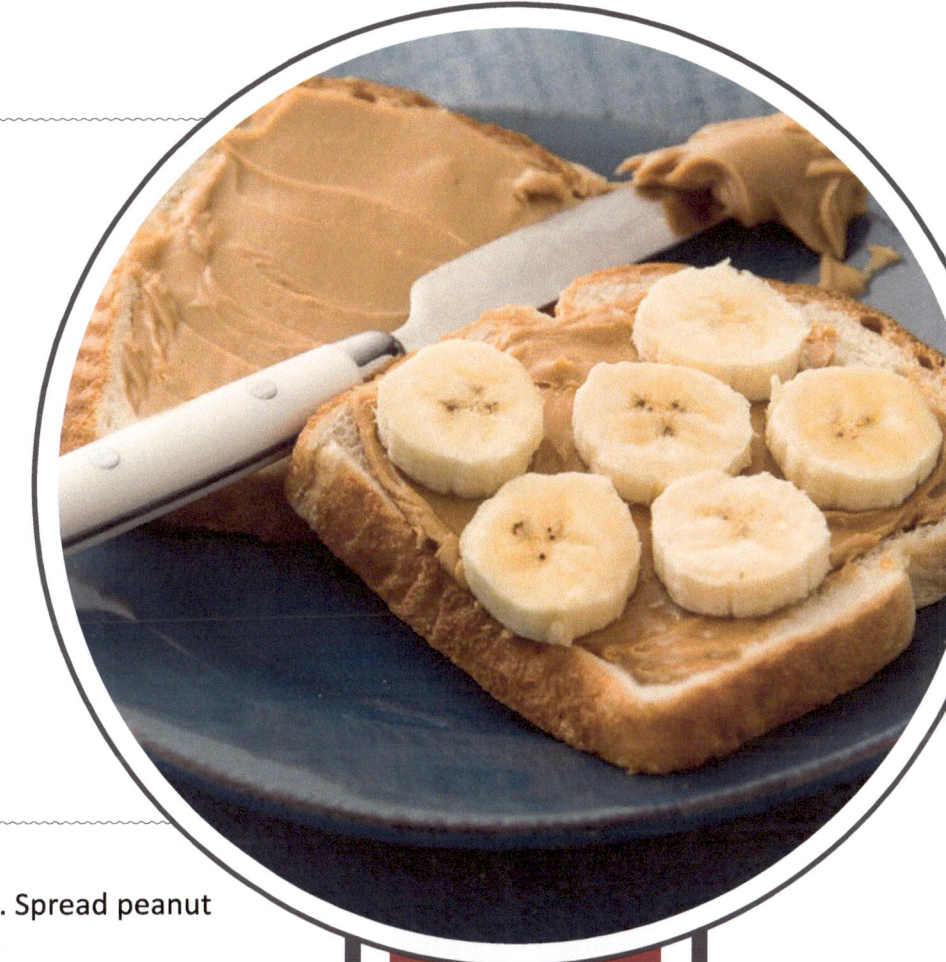

Instructions

1. Toast the bread slice until golden brown. Spread peanut butter smoothly over the toasted bread.
2. Arrange the banana slices on top of the peanut butter. Drizzle honey on top and sprinkle cinnamon powder if desired.
3. Serve immediately and enjoy.

PREP TIME:
10 MINS

COOK TIME:
0 MINS

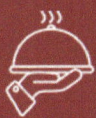

SERVING
2

Nutritional Values (per serving)

Calories: 250, Protein: 8g, Carbohydrates: 35g, Fat: 10g, Fiber: 4g

Cheesy Scrambled Eggs

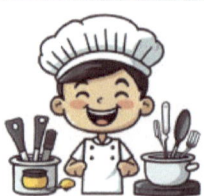

Ingredients

4 large eggs
1/4 cup shredded cheddar cheese
2 tablespoons milk
1 tablespoon butter
Salt and pepper to taste

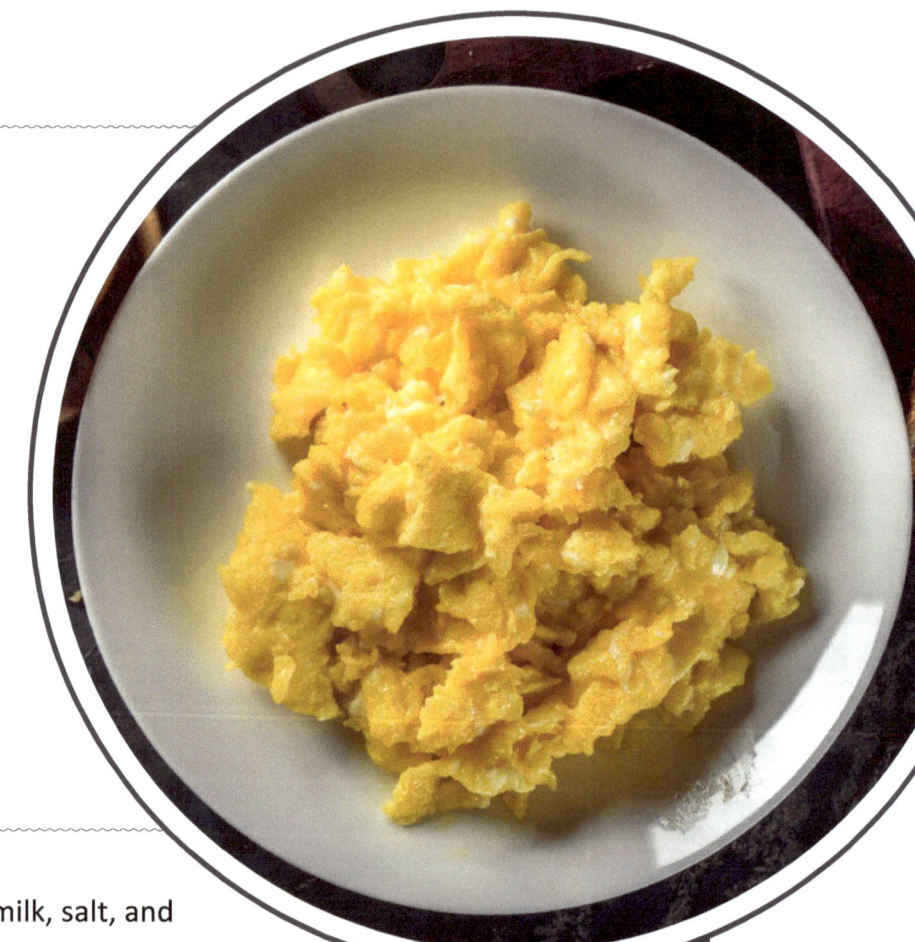

Instructions

1. In a deep-bottom bowl, pulse the eggs, milk, salt, and crushed pepper until well combined.
2. Melt the butter over medium heat.
3. Ladle egg mixture into the skillet and cook, stirring softly, until the eggs begin to set.
4. Sprinkle the shredded cheese over the moderately set eggs and keep cooking until the eggs are fully set and the cheese is melted. Serve immediately and enjoy.

Nutritional Values (per serving)

Calories: 220, Protein: 15g, Carbohydrates: 2g, Fat: 18g, Fiber: 0g

PREP TIME:
10 MINS

COOK TIME:
5 MINS

SERVING
2

Fruit and Yogurt Parfait

Ingredients

1 cup Greek yogurt
1/2 cup mixed berries
1/4 cup granola
1 tablespoon honey (if you want)

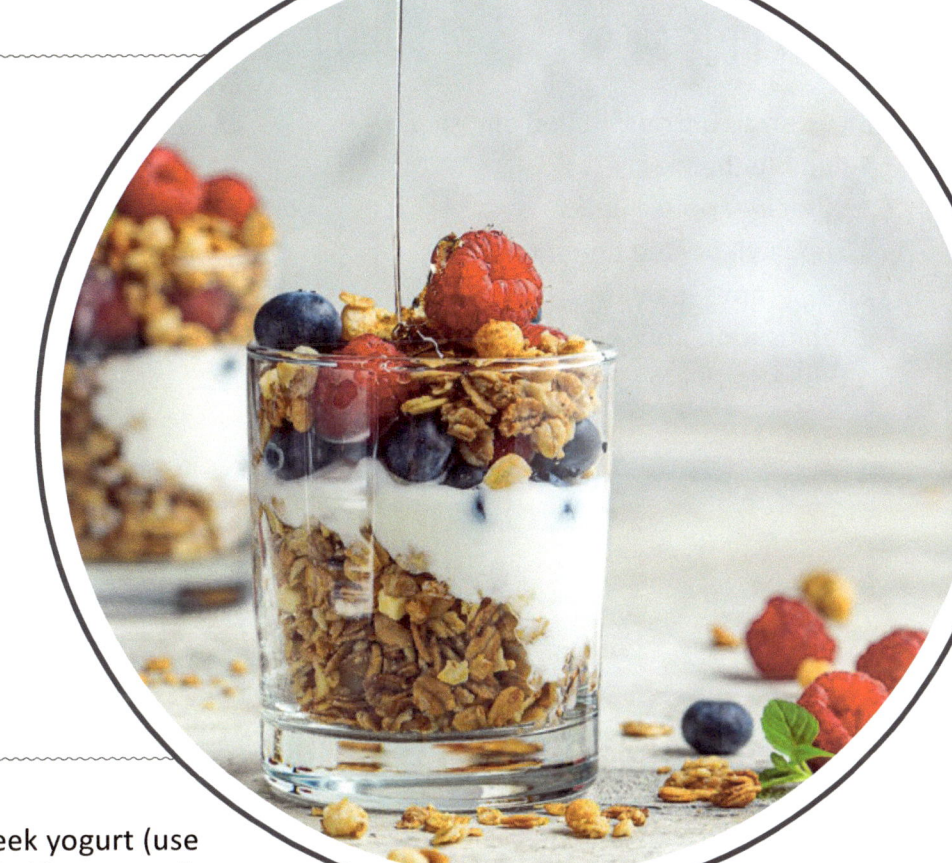

Instructions

1. In a wide-mouth glass or bowl, layer Greek yogurt (use half). Also add mixed berries layer (use half) on top of the yogurt.
2. Sprinkle 1/2 granola over the berries. Repeat the layers with the leftover yogurt, berries, and granola.
3. Drizzle honey on top if desired and serve immediately.

PREP TIME:
10 MINS

COOK TIME:
0 MINS

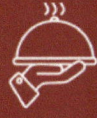

SERVING
2

Nutritional Values (per serving)

Calories: 250, Protein: 14g, Carbohydrates: 35g, Fat: 7g, Fiber: 4g

Rainbow Fruit Salad

Ingredients

1 cup strawberries, hulled and sliced
1 cup blueberries
1 cup pineapple chunks
1 cup kiwi, peeled and sliced
1 cup grapes, halved
1 tablespoon honey (optional)
1 tablespoon lime juice (optional)

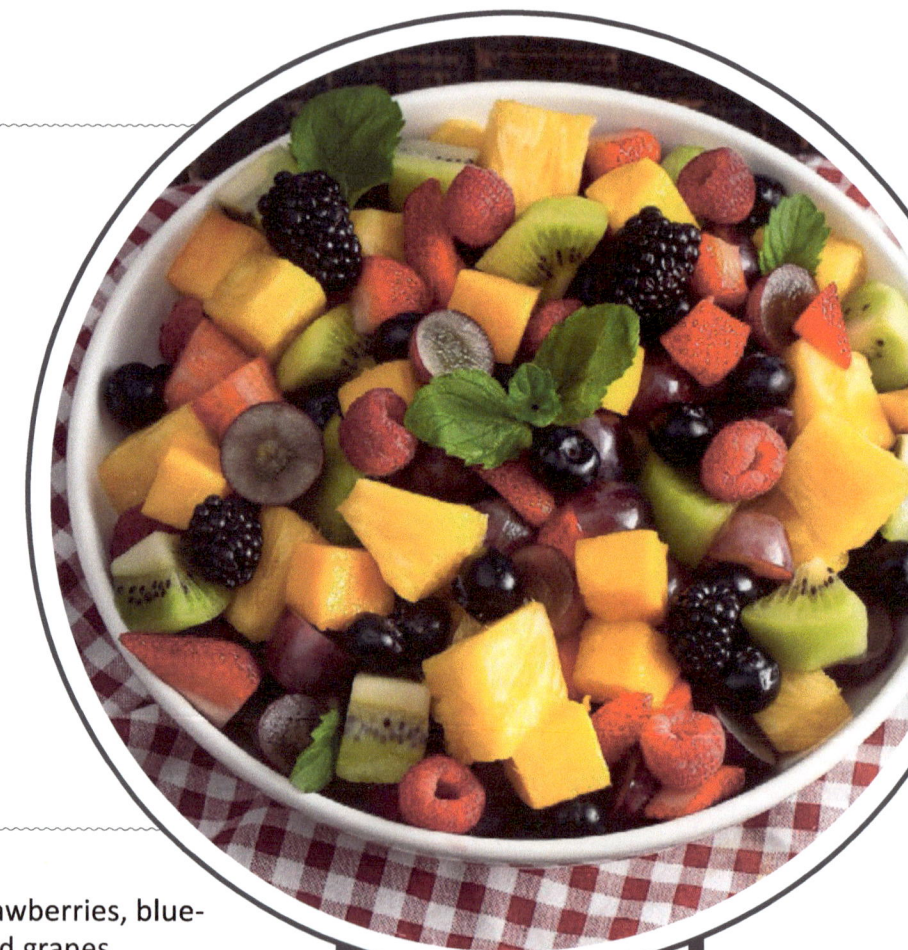

Instructions

1. In a deep-bottom bowl, combine the strawberries, blueberries, pineapple chunks, kiwi slices, and grapes.
2. Drizzle honey and lime juice over the fruit, if desired, and gently toss to combine. Serve immediately or chill before eating.

PREP TIME:
10 MINS

COOK TIME:
0 MINS

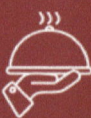

SERVING
2

Nutritional Values (per serving)

Calories: 100, Protein: 1g, Carbohydrates: 26g, Fat: 0g, Fiber: 4g

Cinnamon Toast Sticks

Ingredients

4 slices of bread
2 tablespoons butter, melted
1/4 cup sugar
1 teaspoon cinnamon

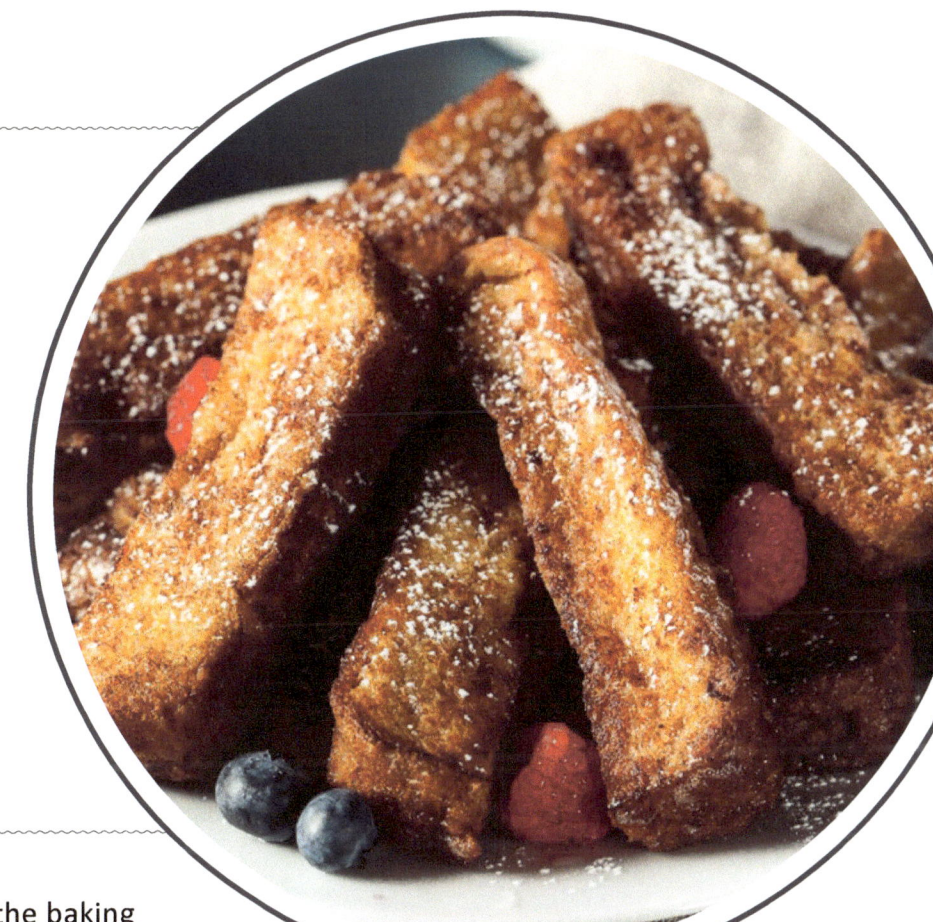

Instructions

1. Preheat oven to 350°F (175°C). Arrange the baking sheet with parchment paper. Cut each slice of bread into three sticks.
2. Mix the sugar and cinnamon in a deep-bottom bowl. Brush the breadsticks with butter and then coat them with the cinnamon-sugar mixture.
3. Arrange the sticks on the baking sheet and bake for 10 minutes.

PREP TIME:
10 MINS

COOK TIME:
5 MINS

SERVING
2

Nutritional Values (per serving)

Calories: 200, Protein: 4g, Carbohydrates: 30g, Fat: 8g, Fiber: 2g

Veggie and Cheese Omelet

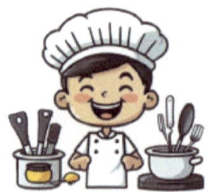

Ingredients

2 large eggs
1/4 cup diced bell peppers
1/4 cup diced tomatoes
1/4 cup shredded cheddar cheese
1 tablespoon butter
Salt and pepper to taste

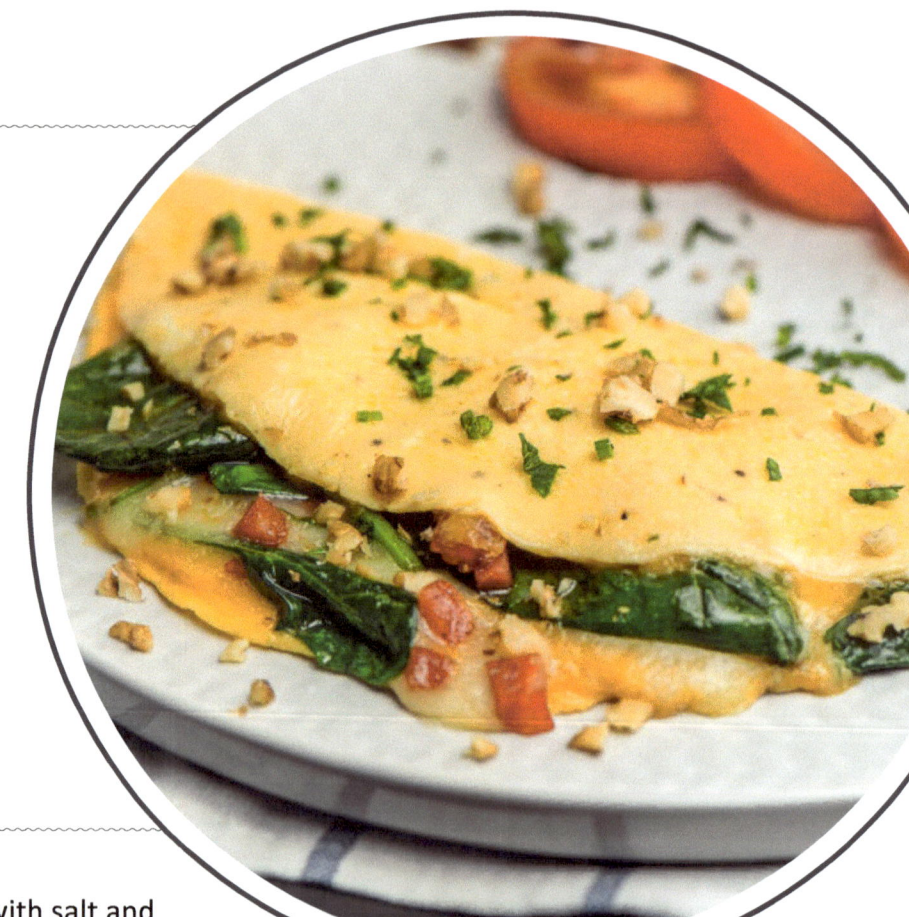

Instructions

1. In a deep-bottom bowl, whisk the eggs with salt and pepper. Melt the butter over medium heat.
2. Ladle eggs into the skillet and cook until they begin to set. Add chopped diced bell peppers and tomatoes evenly over the eggs.
3. Sprinkle shredded cheese to garnish on top and fold the omelet in half. Cook until the cheese is melted and the omelet is fully set.

PREP TIME:
10 MINS

COOK TIME:
5 MINS

SERVING
2

Nutritional Values (per serving)

Calories: 250, Protein: 15g, Carbohydrates: 4g, Fat: 20g, Fiber: 1g

Easy French Toast

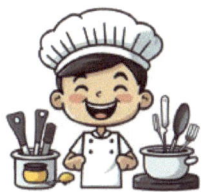

Ingredients

4 slices of bread
2 large eggs
1/2 cup milk
1 teaspoon vanilla extract
1/2 teaspoon cinnamon
2 tablespoons butter

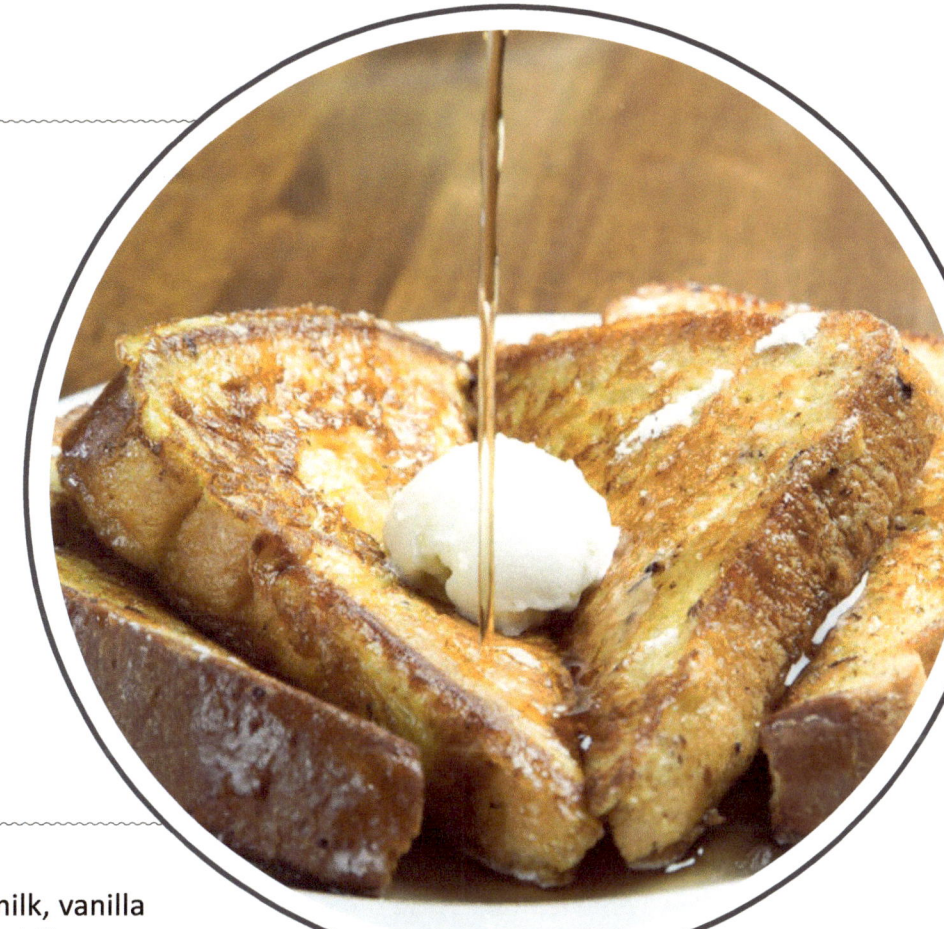

Instructions

1. In a deep-bottom bowl, pulse the eggs, milk, vanilla extract, and cinnamon. Put the non-stick skillet over medium heat and melt the butter.
2. Dip every bread slice into the egg mixture, coating both sides. Place the bread slices and cook until golden brown on both sides, about 2-3 minutes per side.
3. Serve warm with your favorite toppings.

PREP TIME:
10 MINS

COOK TIME:
5 MINS

SERVING
2

Nutritional Values (per serving)

Calories: 300, Protein: 10g, Carbohydrates: 36g, Fat: 14g, Fiber: 2g

Microwave Egg Mug

Ingredients

2 large eggs
2 tablespoons milk
2 tablespoons shredded cheese
Salt and pepper to taste
Optional: diced vegetables (bell peppers, spinach, tomatoes)

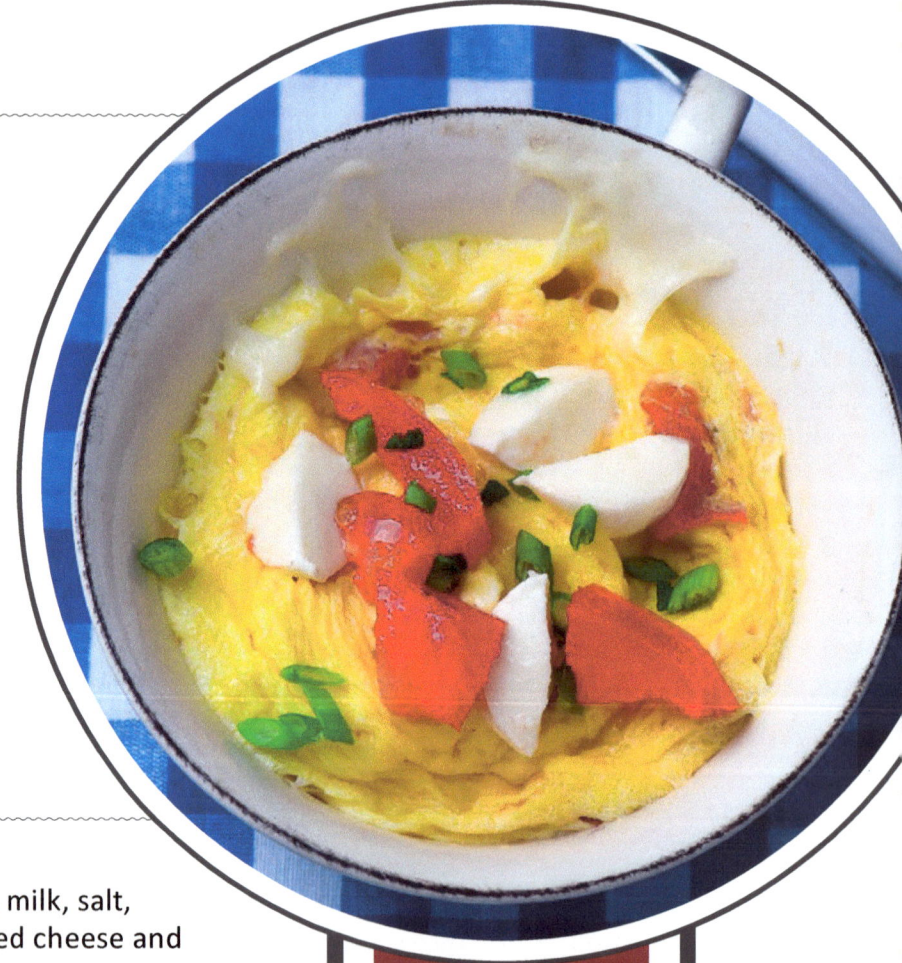

Instructions

1. In a microwave-safe mug, pulse the eggs, milk, salt, and crushed pepper. If using, add shredded cheese and diced vegetables.
2. Microwave on high-heat setting for 1 minute, stir well, and microwave again for 30 seconds minute until the eggs are set.
3. Let it cool slightly before eating directly from the mug.

PREP TIME:
10 MINS

COOK TIME:
5 MINS

SERVING
2

Nutritional Values (per serving)

Calories: 200, Protein: 14g, Carbohydrates: 2g, Fat: 15g, Fiber: 0g

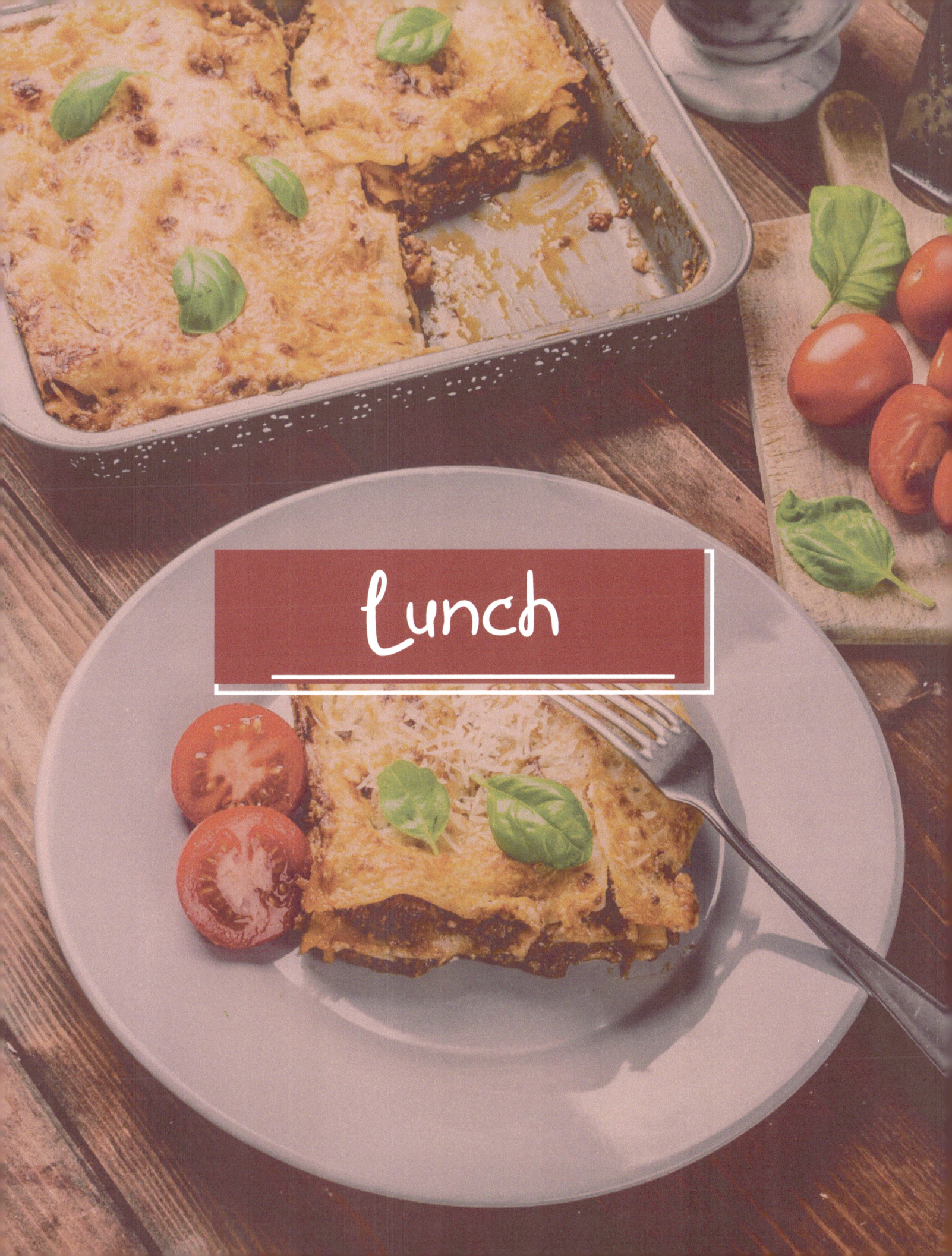

lunch

Mini Pita Pizzas

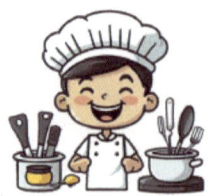

Ingredients

4 mini pita breads
1/2 cup pizza sauce
1 cup shredded mozzarella cheese
1/2 cup sliced bell peppers
1/4 cup sliced olives

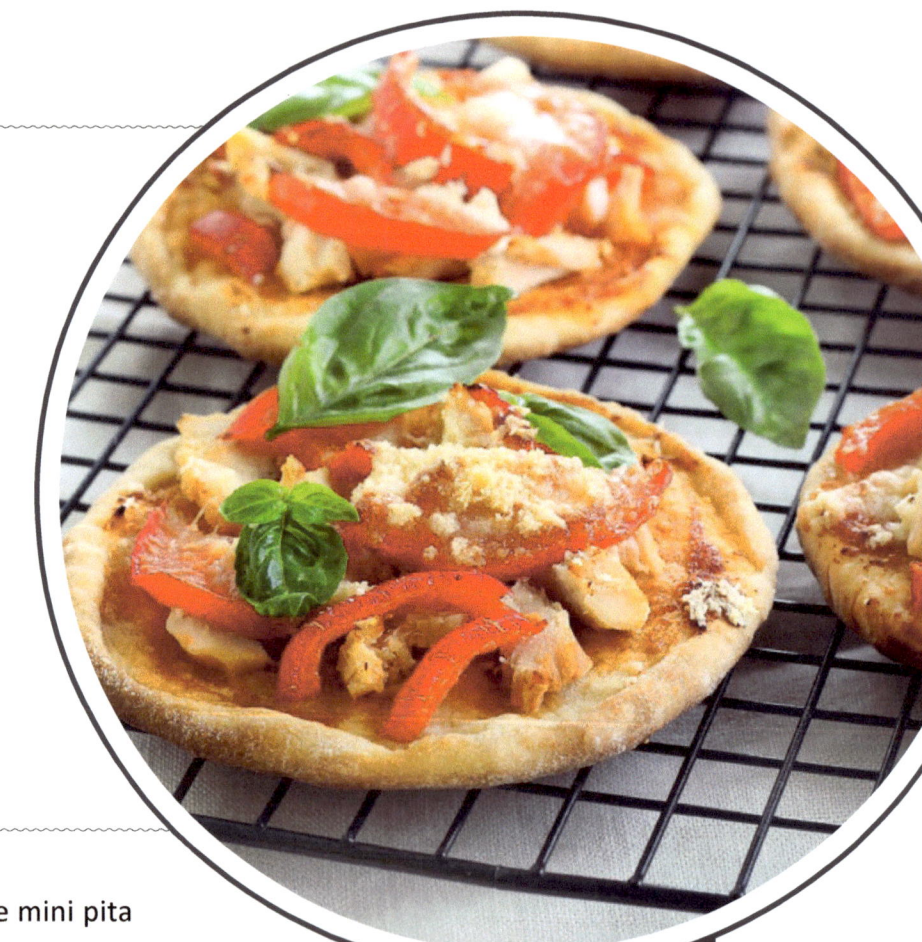

Instructions

1. Preheat oven to 375°F (190°C). Place the mini pita breads on a baking sheet.
2. Spread pizza sauce evenly on each pita bread. Sprinkle shredded mozzarella cheese on top.
3. Add sliced bell peppers and olives. Bake for 10 minutes.

PREP TIME:
10 MINS

COOK TIME:
10 MINS

SERVING
2

Nutritional Values (per serving)

Calories: 250, Protein: 12g, Carbohydrates: 30g, Fat: 10g, Fiber: 2g

Colorful Veggie Wraps

Ingredients

2 large whole wheat tortillas
1/2 cup hummus
1/2 cup shredded carrots
1/2 cup sliced bell peppers
1/2 cup spinach leaves
1/4 cup sliced cucumbers

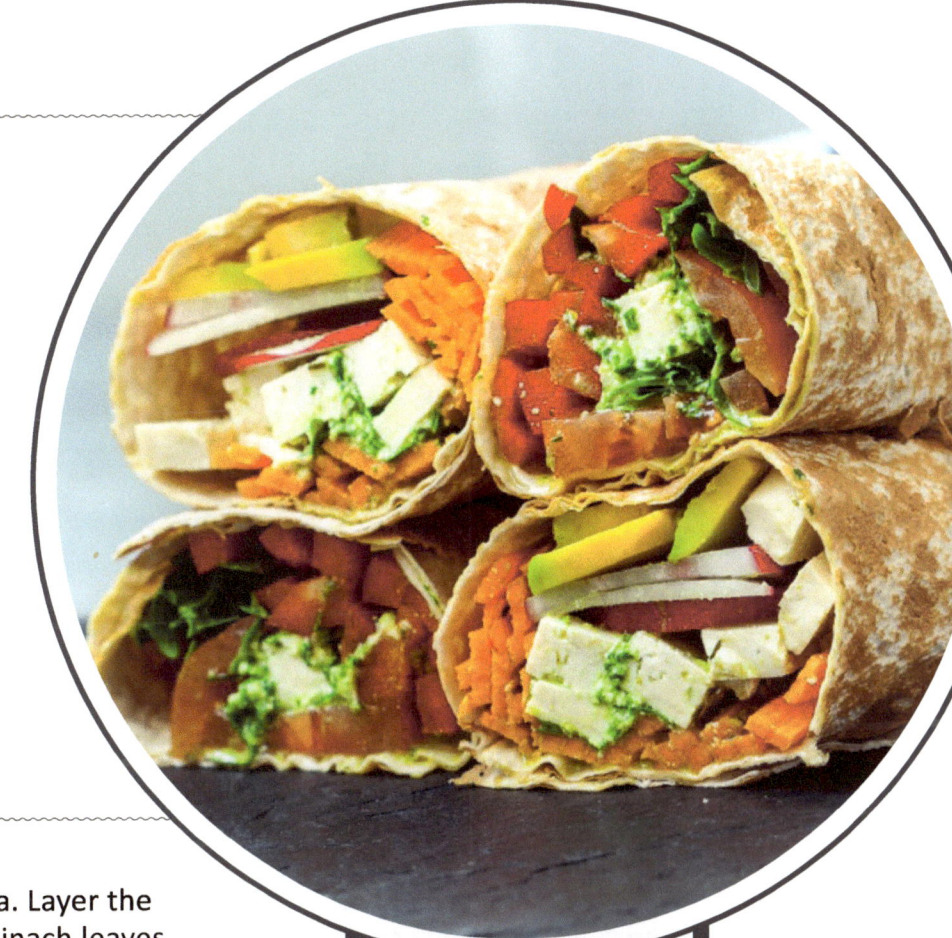

Instructions

1. Spread hummus evenly over each tortilla. Layer the shredded carrots, sliced bell peppers, spinach leaves, and sliced cucumbers on top.
2. Roll up the tortillas tightly. Cut the wraps in half and serve immediately.

PREP TIME:
10 MINS

COOK TIME:
0 MINS

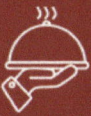

SERVING
2

Nutritional Values (per serving)

Calories: 200, Protein: 6g, Carbohydrates: 30g, Fat: 8g, Fiber: 6g

Chicken Salad Sandwiches

Ingredients

1 cup cooked chicken, diced
1/4 cup mayonnaise
1/4 cup diced celery
1 tablespoon lemon juice
Salt and pepper to taste
4 slices whole grain bread

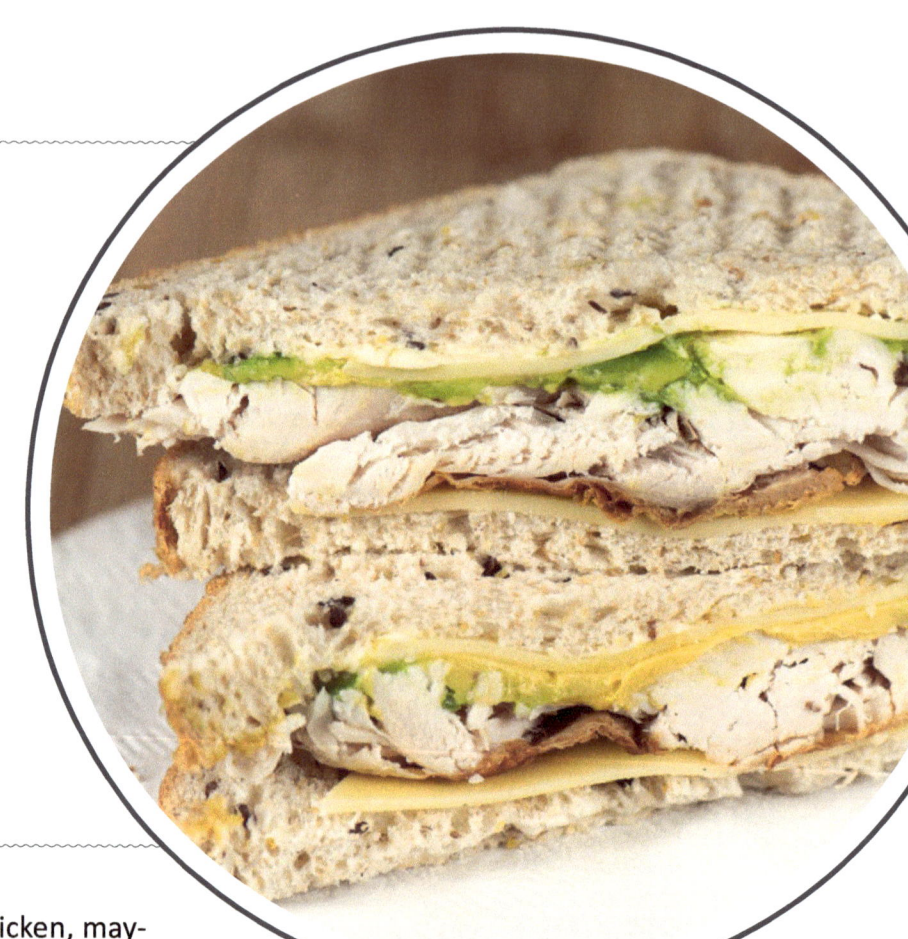

Instructions

1. In a deep-bottom bowl, mix the diced chicken, mayonnaise, diced celery, lemon juice, salt, and crushed pepper until well combined.
2. Spread the chicken salad mixture evenly over two slices of bread. Top with slices of leftover bread to form sandwiches. Cut the sandwiches in half and serve.

PREP TIME:
10 MINS

COOK TIME:
0 MINS

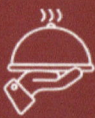

SERVING
2

Nutritional Values (per serving)

Calories: 350, Protein: 20g, Carbohydrates: 32g, Fat: 16g, Fiber: 4g

Easy Cheesy Quesadillas

Ingredients

2 large flour tortillas
1 cup shredded cheddar cheese
1/2 cup salsa (optional)

Add if desired:
1/2 cup cooked and chopped meat (chicken, beef, pork,etc)

Instructions

1. Put the non-stick skillet over medium flame. Place one tortilla and sprinkle the shredded cheddar cheese evenly over it. Add meat (if desired) evenly across the tortilla.
2. Place the second tortilla on top of the cheese. Cook for 2-3 minutes on one side until the cheese melts properly and the tortillas are golden brown. Cut into wedges and take it with salsa if desired.

PREP TIME:
10 MINS

COOK TIME:
5 MINS

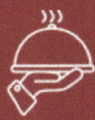

SERVING
2

Nutritional Values (per serving)

Calories: 300, Protein: 14g, Carbohydrates: 28g, Fat: 16g, Fiber: 2g

Turkey and Cheese Roll-Ups

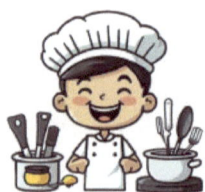

Ingredients

4 slices of turkey breast
4 slices of cheddar cheese
2 whole wheat tortillas
1/4 cup baby spinach leaves

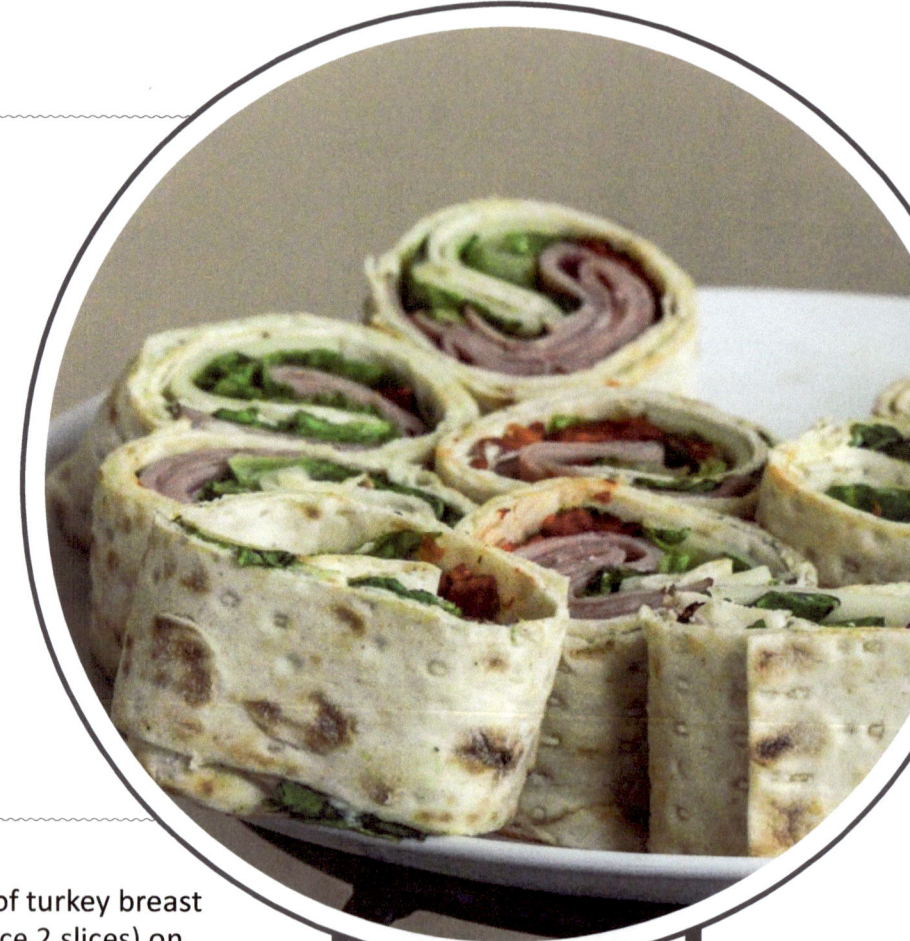

Instructions

1. Lay the tortillas flat and place two slices of turkey breast on each. Place cheddar cheese slices (place 2 slices) on top of the turkey.
2. Sprinkle baby spinach leaves over the cheese. Roll up the tortillas tightly, slice each roll-up in half, and serve.

PREP TIME:
10 MINS

COOK TIME:
0 MINS

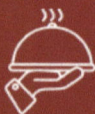

SERVING
2

Nutritional Values (per serving)

Calories: 250, Protein: 20g, Carbohydrates: 18g, Fat: 12g, Fiber: 2g

Veggie Pasta Salad

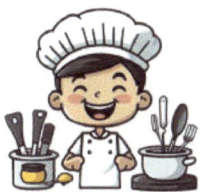

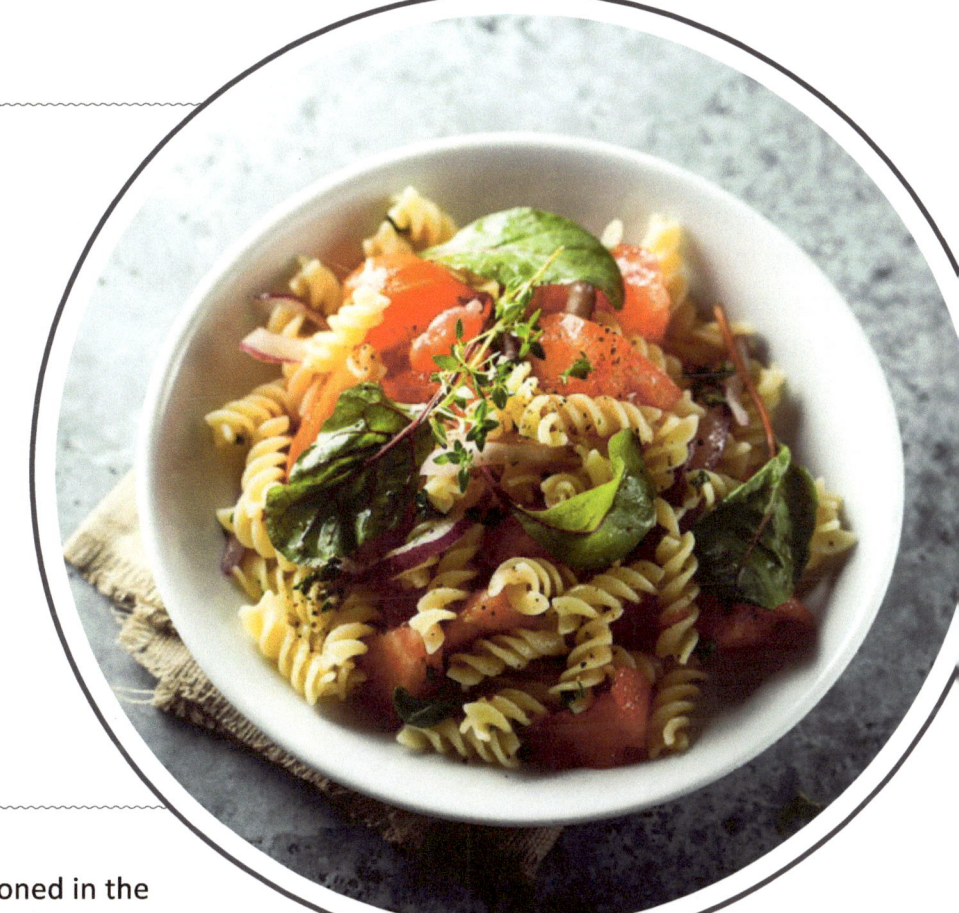

Ingredients

2 cups cooked pasta (rotini or penne)
1 cup cherry tomatoes, halved
1/2 cup diced cucumber
1/2 cup diced bell peppers
1/4 cup sliced black olives
1/4 cup Italian dressing

Instructions

1. Cook pasta according to the steps mentioned in the packet guidelines, then drain and let it cool.
2. In a deep-bottom bowl, combine the cooked pasta, cherry tomatoes, diced cucumber, diced bell peppers, and sliced black olives.
3. Drop Italian dressing over the salad and toss to coat. Chill in the refrigerator for thirty minutes (at least) before serving.

PREP TIME:
10 MINS

COOK TIME:
10 MINS

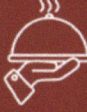

SERVING
2

Nutritional Values (per serving)

Calories: 200, Protein: 5g, Carbohydrates: 30g, Fat: 8g, Fiber: 2g

MAC AND CHEESE BITES

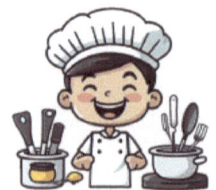

INGREDIENTS

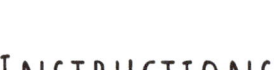

2 cups cooked macaroni
1 cup shredded cheddar cheese
1/2 cup milk
1 large egg, beaten
1/4 cup breadcrumbs

INSTRUCTIONS

1. Preheat oven to 375°F (190°C). Grease a mini muffin tin. In a deep-bottom bowl, mix the cooked macaroni, shredded cheddar cheese, milk, and beaten egg until well combined.
2. Spoon the macaroni mixture into the mini muffin tin, filling each cup. Sprinkle breadcrumbs on top of each mac and cheese bite.
3. Bake for 15 minutes or until golden brown. Let cool slightly before serving.

PREP TIME:
10 MINS

COOK TIME:
15 MINS

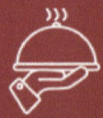

SERVING
2

NUTRITIONAL VALUES (PER SERVING)

Calories: 250, Protein: 10g, Carbohydrates: 30g, Fat: 10g, Fiber: 1g

Rainbow Veggie Sushi Rolls

Ingredients

2 nori sheets
1 cup cooked sushi rice
1/4 cup julienned carrots
1/4 cup julienned cucumber
1/4 cup julienned bell peppers
1/4 cup avocado slices

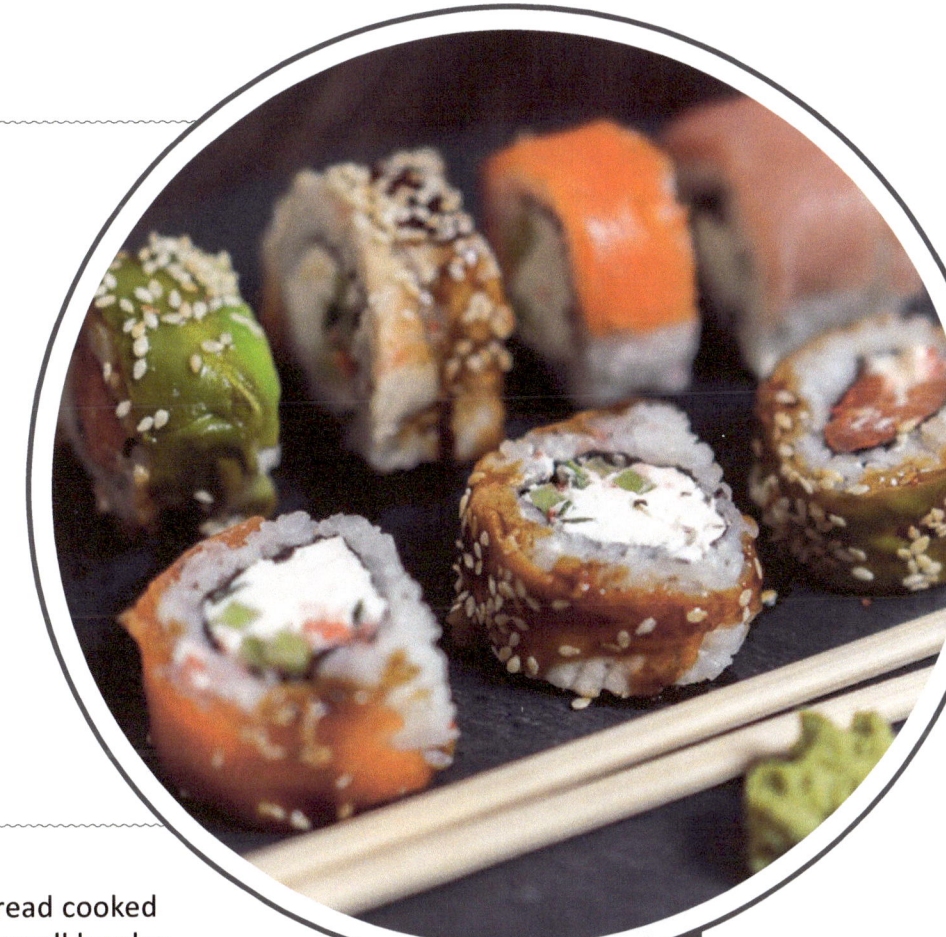

Instructions

1. Place a nori sheet on a clean surface. Spread cooked sushi rice (a thin layer) on top, leaving a small border.
2. Arrange the julienned carrots, cucumber, bell peppers, and avocado slices in a line across the middle of the rice.
3. Roll the nori tightly around the vegetables, using the mat to help if needed. Seal the edge with a little water.
4. Slice the roll into small pieces and serve.

PREP TIME:
10 MINS

COOK TIME:
0 MINS

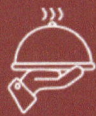

SERVING
2

Nutritional Values (per serving)

Calories: 200, Protein: 4g, Carbohydrates: 40g, Fat: 4g, Fiber: 4g

Caprese Salad Skewers

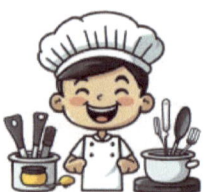

Ingredients

1 cup cherry tomatoes
1 cup mini mozzarella balls
1/4 cup fresh basil leaves
2 tablespoons balsamic glaze
2 tablespoons olive oil
Salt and pepper to taste

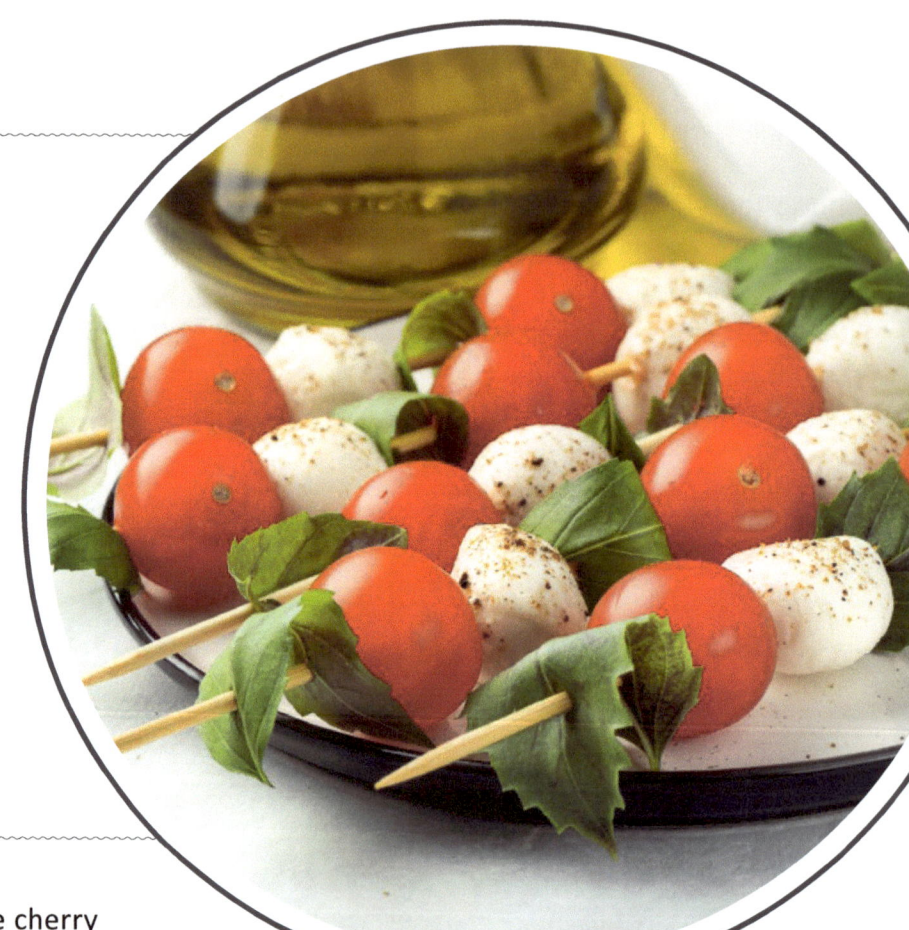

Instructions

1. On small skewers or toothpicks, alternate cherry tomatoes, mini mozzarella balls, and fresh basil leaves.
2. Arrange the skewers on a serving platter. Drizzle with balsamic glaze and olive oil. Sprinkle with salt and pepper to taste. Serve immediately.

PREP TIME:
10 MINS

COOK TIME:
0 MINS

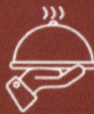

SERVING
4

Nutritional Values (per serving)

Calories: 150, Protein: 6g, Carbohydrates: 4g, Fat: 12g, Fiber: 1g

Cheesy Broccoli Bites

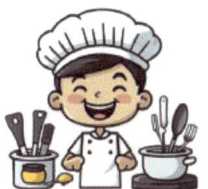

Ingredients

2 cups broccoli florets, steamed and chopped
1 cup shredded cheddar cheese
1/2 cup breadcrumbs
1 large egg, beaten
1/2 teaspoon garlic powder
Salt and pepper to taste

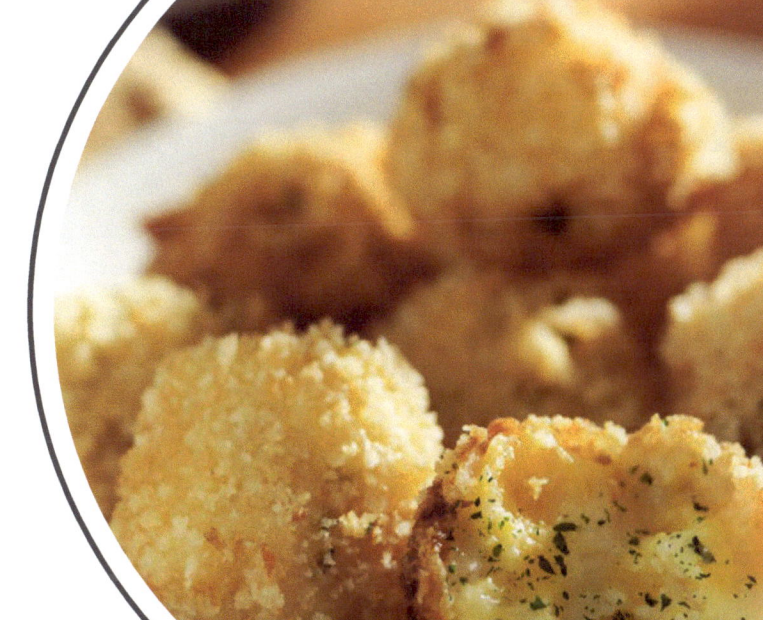

Instructions

1. Preheat oven to 375°F (190°C). Arrange the baking sheet with parchment paper.
2. In a deep-bottom bowl, mix the chopped broccoli, shredded cheddar cheese, breadcrumbs, beaten egg, garlic powder, salt, and crushed pepper until well combined.
3. Scoop out small portions of the mixture and form into bite-sized balls or patties. Place the broccoli bites on the prepared baking sheet.
4. Bake for 12-15 minutes. Let cool slightly before serving.

PREP TIME:
10 MINS

COOK TIME:
15 MINS

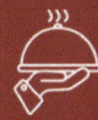

SERVING
2

Nutritional Values (per serving)

Calories: 180, Protein: 10g, Carbohydrates: 15g, Fat: 9g, Fiber: 3g

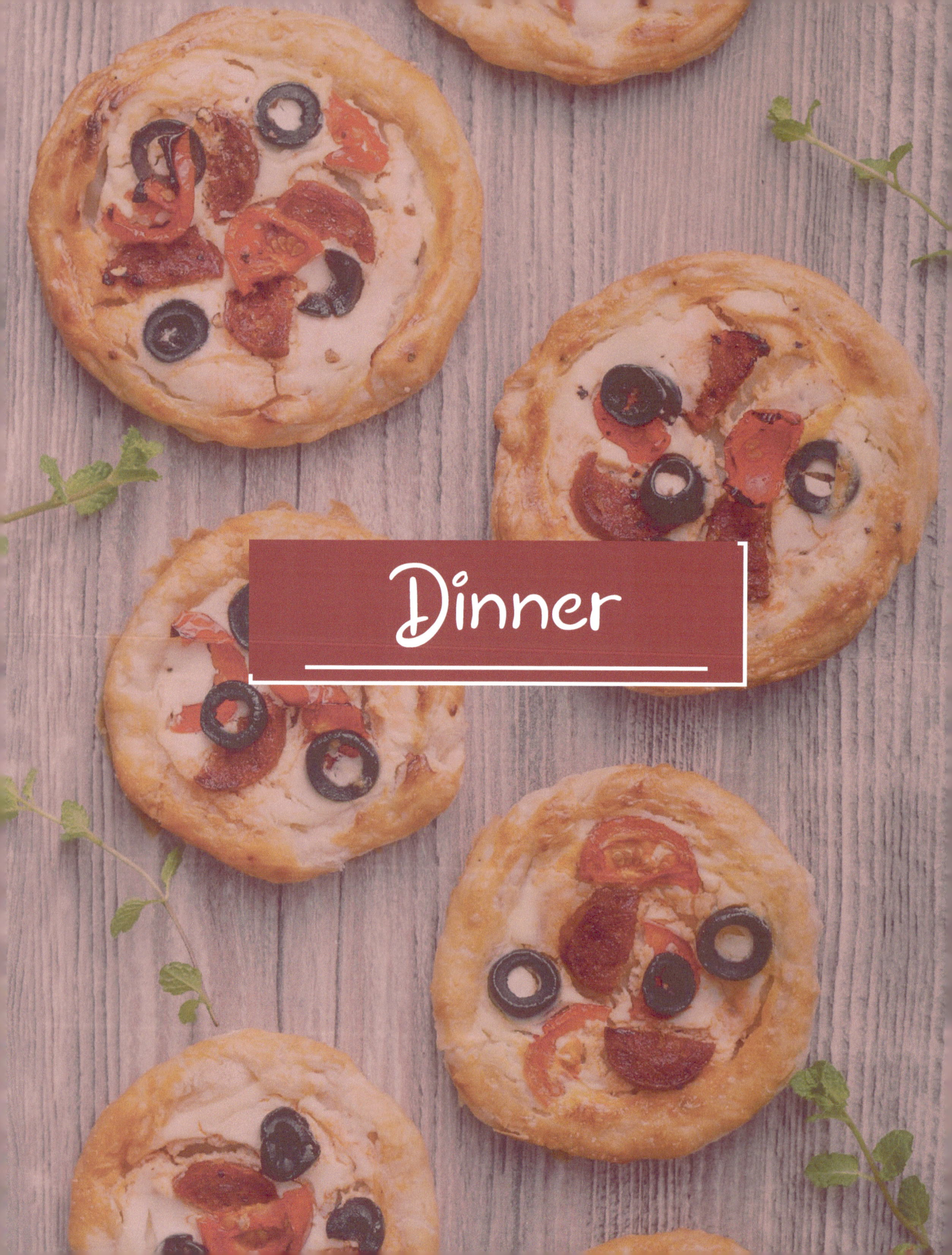

Dinner

Spaghetti and Meatballs

Ingredients

8 oz spaghetti
1 cup marinara sauce
1/2 lb ground beef
1/4 cup breadcrumbs
1/4 cup grated Parmesan cheese
1 large egg
1/2 teaspoon garlic powder
Salt and pepper to taste

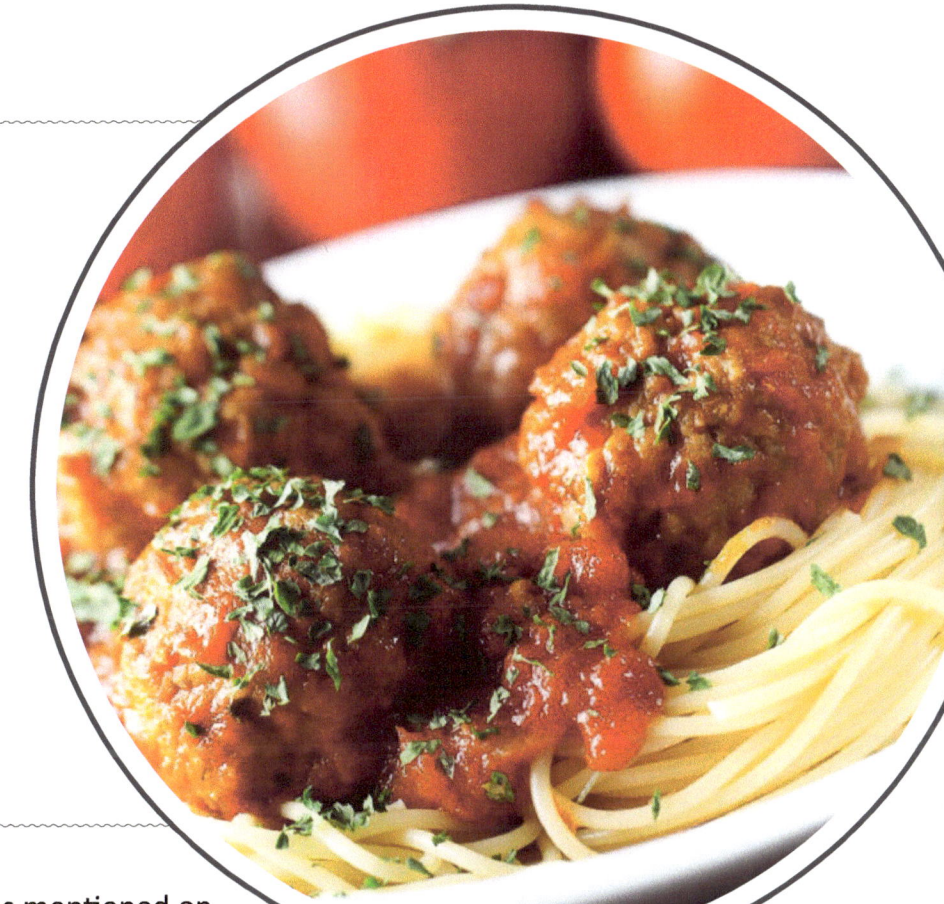

Instructions

1. Cook the spaghetti according to the steps mentioned on the packet guidelines. Drain and set aside.
2. In a deep-bottom bowl, mix the ground beef, breadcrumbs, Parmesan cheese, egg, garlic powder, salt, and crushed pepper. Form into small meatballs.
3. In a skillet, cook the meatballs over medium flame until browned on all sides, about 10 minutes.
4. Add marinara sauce and simmer for another 10 minutes. Serve the meatballs with sauce over the prepared spaghetti.

PREP TIME:
10 MINS

COOK TIME:
25 MINS

SERVING
4

Nutritional Values (per serving)

Calories: 400, Protein: 20g, Carbohydrates: 45g, Fat: 15g, Fiber: 3g

MINI TURKEY BURGERS

INGREDIENTS

1 lb ground turkey

1/4 cup breadcrumbs

1/4 cup grated onion

1 large egg

1/2 teaspoon garlic powder

Salt and pepper to taste

4 mini burger buns

Lettuce, tomato, and cheese slices for serving

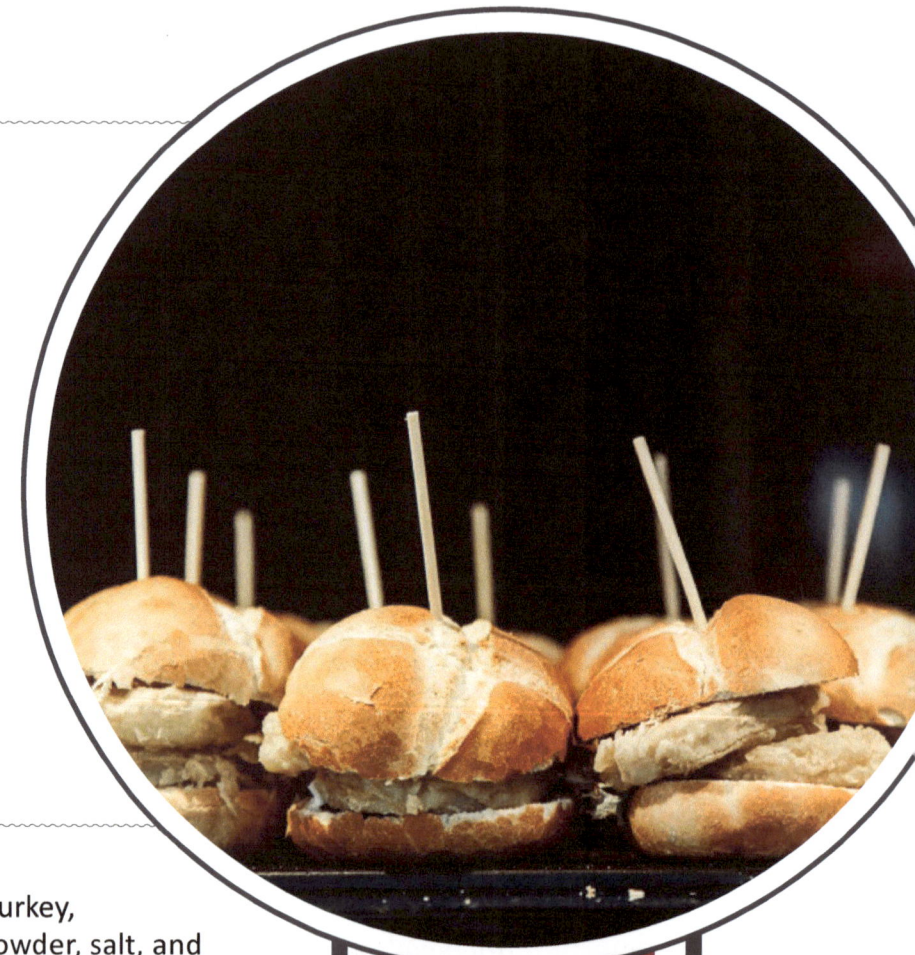

INSTRUCTIONS

1. In a deep-bottom bowl, mix the ground turkey, breadcrumbs, grated onion, egg, garlic powder, salt, and crushed pepper. Form into small patties.
2. Put the non-stick skillet over medium heat and cook the turkey patties for 5 minutes on one side or until fully cooked.
3. Toast the mini burger buns in the skillet if desired. Assemble the mini burgers with lettuce, tomato, and cheese slices. Serve immediately.

PREP TIME:
10 MINS

COOK TIME:
10 MINS

SERVING
2

NUTRITIONAL VALUES (PER SERVING)

Calories: 300, Protein: 20g, Carbohydrates: 25g, Fat: 12g, Fiber: 2g

Homemade Chicken Nuggets

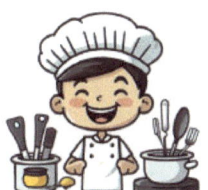

Ingredients

1 lb. chicken breast, cut into pieces
1 cup breadcrumbs
1/2 cup grated Parmesan cheese
1 large egg, beaten
1/4 cup flour
Salt and pepper to taste

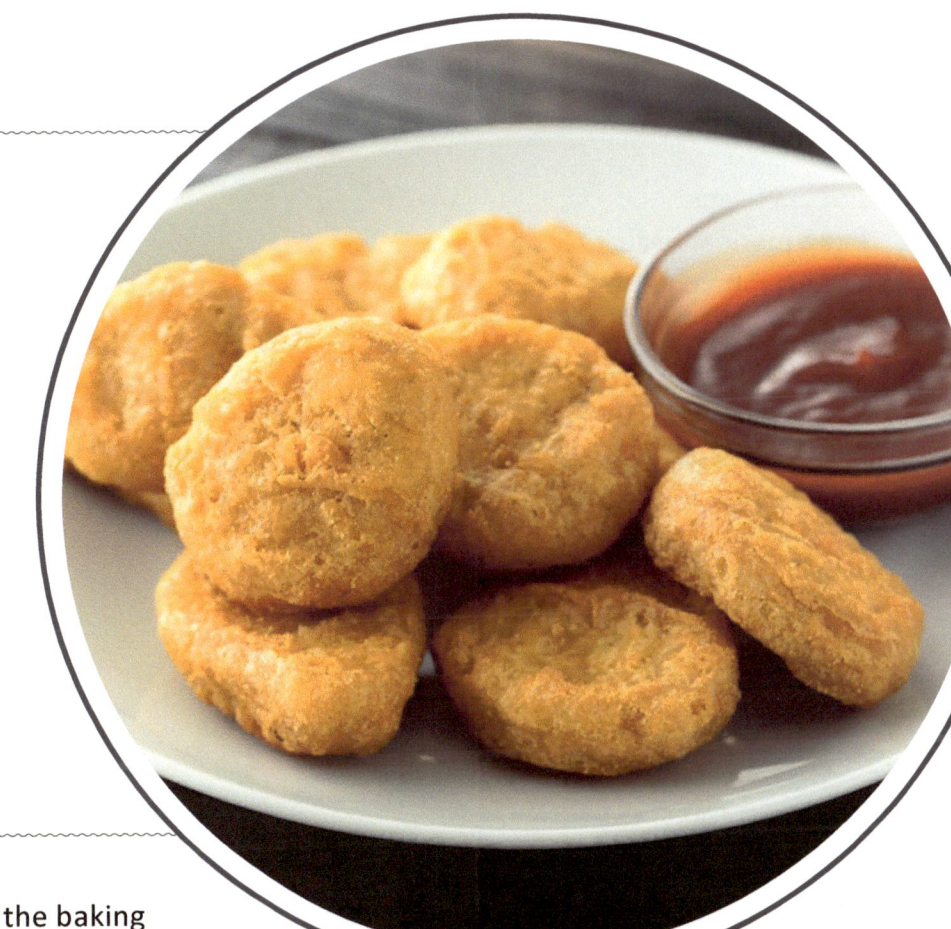

Instructions

1. Preheat oven to 400°F (200°C). Arrange the baking sheet with parchment paper. Powder the chicken pieces with salt and pepper.
2. Dredge every piece in flour, then dip in the pulsed egg and coat with the breadcrumbs and Parmesan cheese mixture. Place the coated chicken nuggets on the prepared baking sheet.
3. Bake for 15 minutes until golden brown and fully cooked. Serve with your favorite dipping sauce.

PREP TIME:
10 MINS

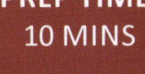

COOK TIME:
25 MINS

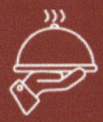

SERVING
4

Nutritional Values (per serving)

Calories: 250, Protein: 28g, Carbohydrates: 15g, Fat: 10g, Fiber: 1g

Cheesy Baked Ziti

Ingredients

8 oz ziti pasta
1 cup marinara sauce
1 cup ricotta cheese
1 cup shredded mozzarella cheese
1/4 cup grated Parmesan cheese
1 teaspoon dried basil
Salt and pepper to taste

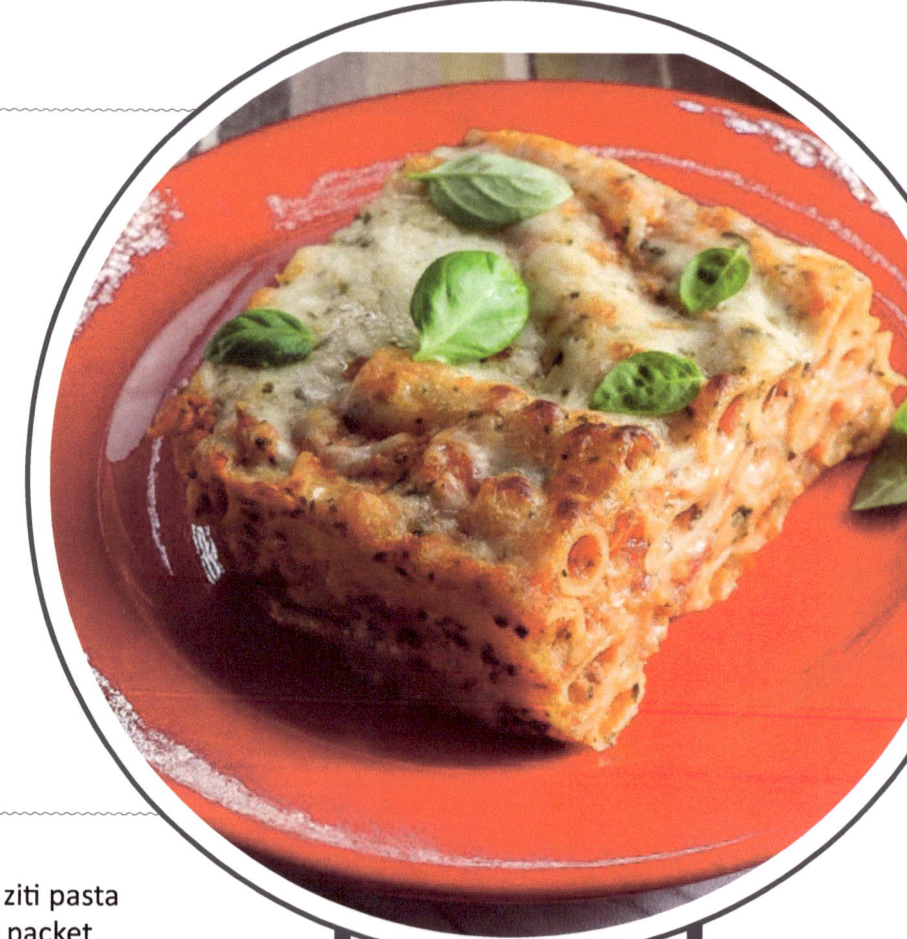

Instructions

1. Preheat oven to 375°F (190°C). Cook the ziti pasta according to the steps mentioned on the packet guidelines. Drain and set aside.
2. In a deep-bottom bowl, mix the cooked pasta with marinara sauce, ricotta cheese, and half of the shredded mozzarella cheese. Season with dried basil, salt, and crushed pepper.
3. Shift the pasta mixture to the baking dish and top with the leftover mozzarella cheese and grated Parmesan cheese.
4. Bake for 22-25 minutes until the cheese melts properly and bubbly. Let cool slightly before serving.

PREP TIME:
10 MINS

COOK TIME:
25 MINS

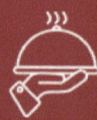

SERVING
4

Nutritional Values (per serving)

Calories: 400, Protein: 20g, Carbohydrates: 50g, Fat: 15g, Fiber: 3g

CHICKEN AND VEGGIE STIR-FRY

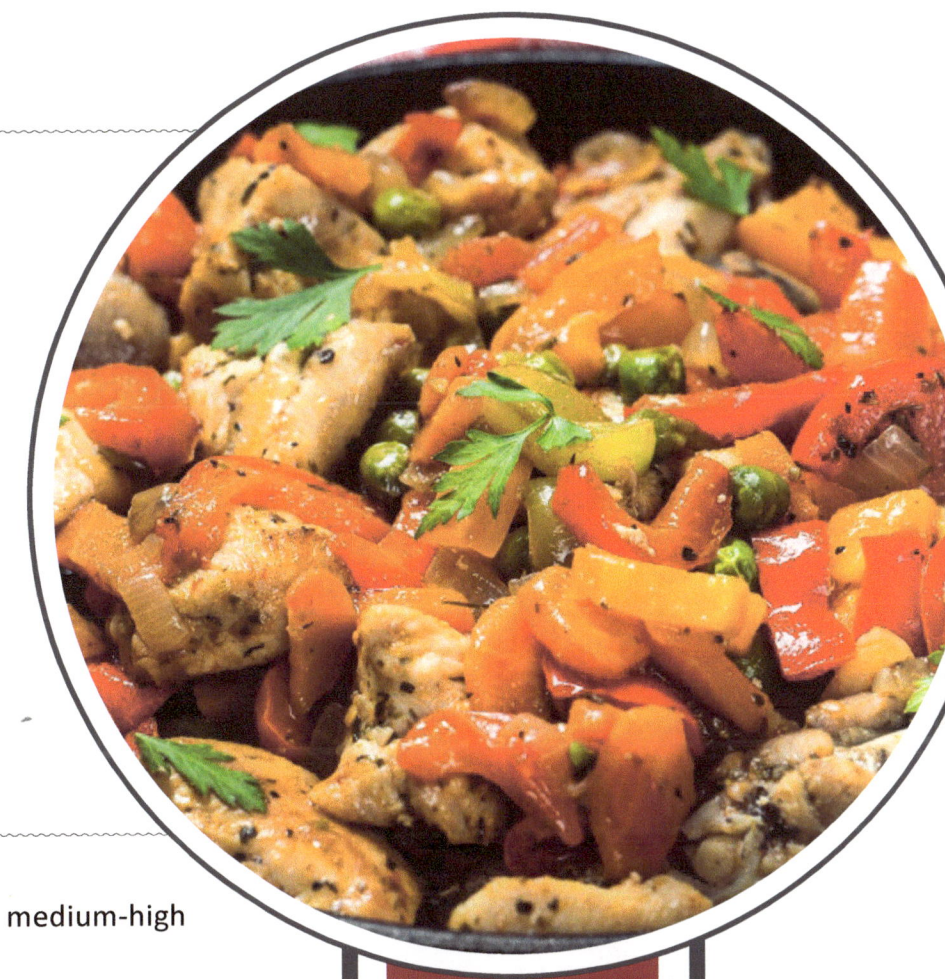

INGREDIENTS

1 lb chicken breast, cut into strips

2 cups mixed vegetables (bell peppers, broccoli, carrots)

2 tablespoons soy sauce

1 tablespoon olive oil

1 teaspoon garlic powder

1 teaspoon ginger powder

1 tablespoon cornstarch pulsed with 2 tablespoons water

INSTRUCTIONS

1. Heat one tbsp oil In a skillet or wok over medium-high heat.
2. Add meat strips and cook until browned and fully cooked, about 5-7 minutes.
3. Add the mixed vegetables, garlic powder, and ginger powder. Fry for another 5 minutes, and keep stirring until the vegetables are tender.
4. Pour in the soy sauce and the cornstarch mixture, stirring until the sauce thickens.
5. Serve immediately over rice or noodles.

PREP TIME:
10 MINS

COOK TIME:
15 MINS

SERVING
4

NUTRITIONAL VALUES (PER SERVING)

Calories: 250, Protein: 25g, Carbohydrates: 10g, Fat: 10g, Fiber: 3g

CREAMY TOMATO PASTA

INGREDIENTS

8 oz pasta (penne or fusilli)
1 cup marinara sauce
1/2 cup heavy cream
1/4 cup grated Parmesan cheese
1 tablespoon olive oil
1 teaspoon garlic powder
Salt and pepper to taste

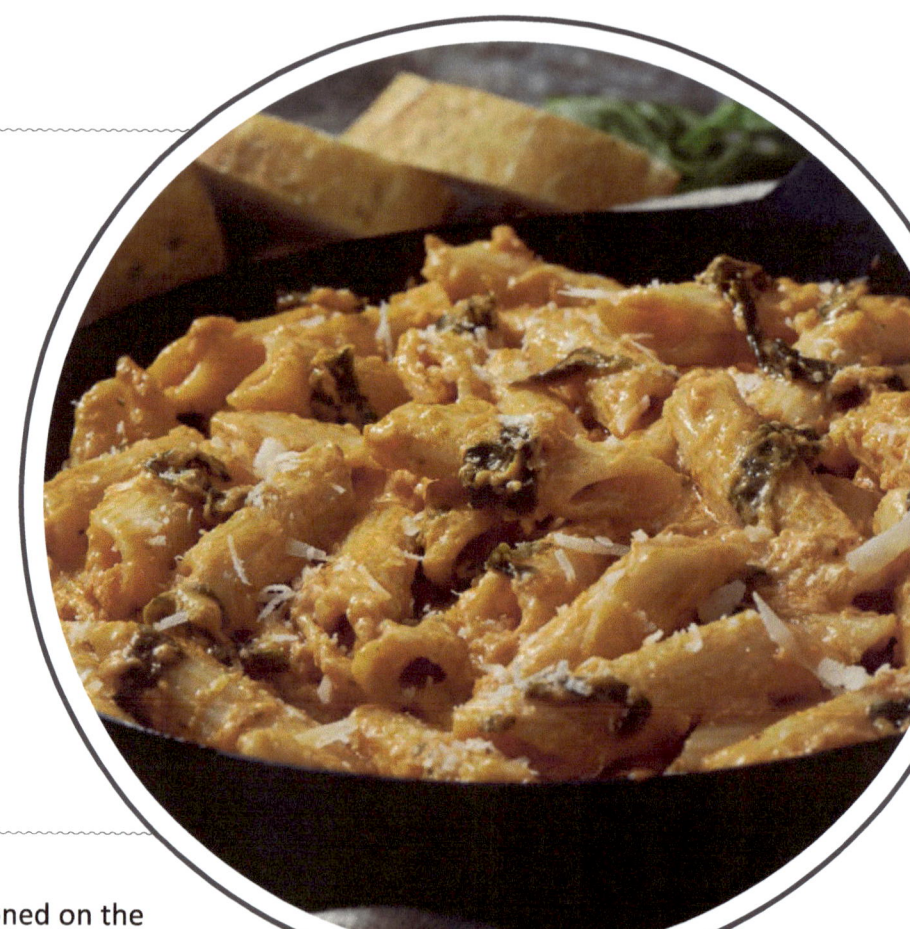

INSTRUCTIONS

1. Cook pasta according to the steps mentioned on the packet guidelines. Drain and set aside.
2. In a skillet, heat one tbsp oil over medium heat. Add the marinara sauce and garlic powder.
3. Add heavy cream, stir it thoroughly and bring to a simmer. Cook for 5 minutes.
4. Add prepared pasta and grated Parmesan cheese to the skillet, tossing to coat evenly.
5. Powder it with salt and crushed pepper to taste. Serve immediately.

PREP TIME:
10 MINS

COOK TIME:
15 MINS

SERVING
4

NUTRITIONAL VALUES (PER SERVING)

Calories: 350, Protein: 10g, Carbohydrates: 45g, Fat: 15g, Fiber: 3g

Baked Fish Sticks

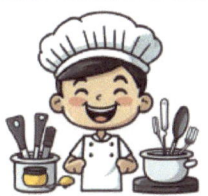

Ingredients

1 lb. white fish any, cut into strips
1 cup breadcrumbs
1/4 cup grated Parmesan cheese
1 large egg, beaten
1/4 cup flour
Salt and pepper to taste

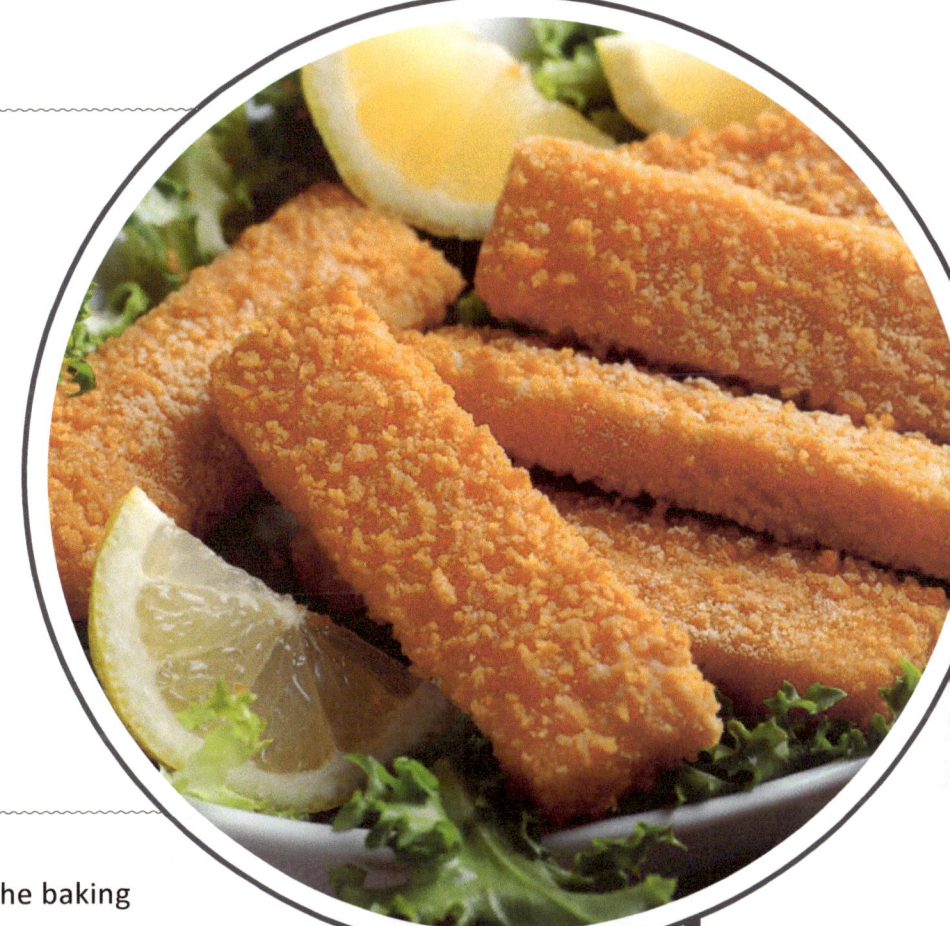

Instructions

1. Preheat oven to 400°F (200°C). Arrange the baking sheet with parchment paper.
2. Powder the fish strips with salt and pepper. Dredge each strip in flour, then dip in the pulsed egg and coat with the breadcrumb and Parmesan cheese mixture.
3. Place the coated fish sticks on the prepared baking sheet.
4. Bake for 12-15 minutes until golden brown and crispy.
5. Serve with your favorite dipping sauce.

PREP TIME:
10 MINS

COOK TIME:
15 MINS

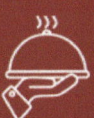

SERVING
4

Nutritional Values (per serving)

Calories: 250, Protein: 25g, Carbohydrates: 10g, Fat: 10g, Fiber: 3g

MINI SHEPHERD'S PIES

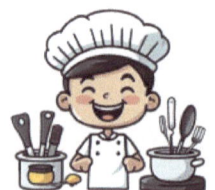

INGREDIENTS

1 lb ground beef
1 cup frozen vegetables, mixed (peas, carrots, corn)
1 cup beef broth
2 tablespoons tomato paste
4 cups mashed potatoes
1 tablespoon olive oil
Salt and pepper to taste

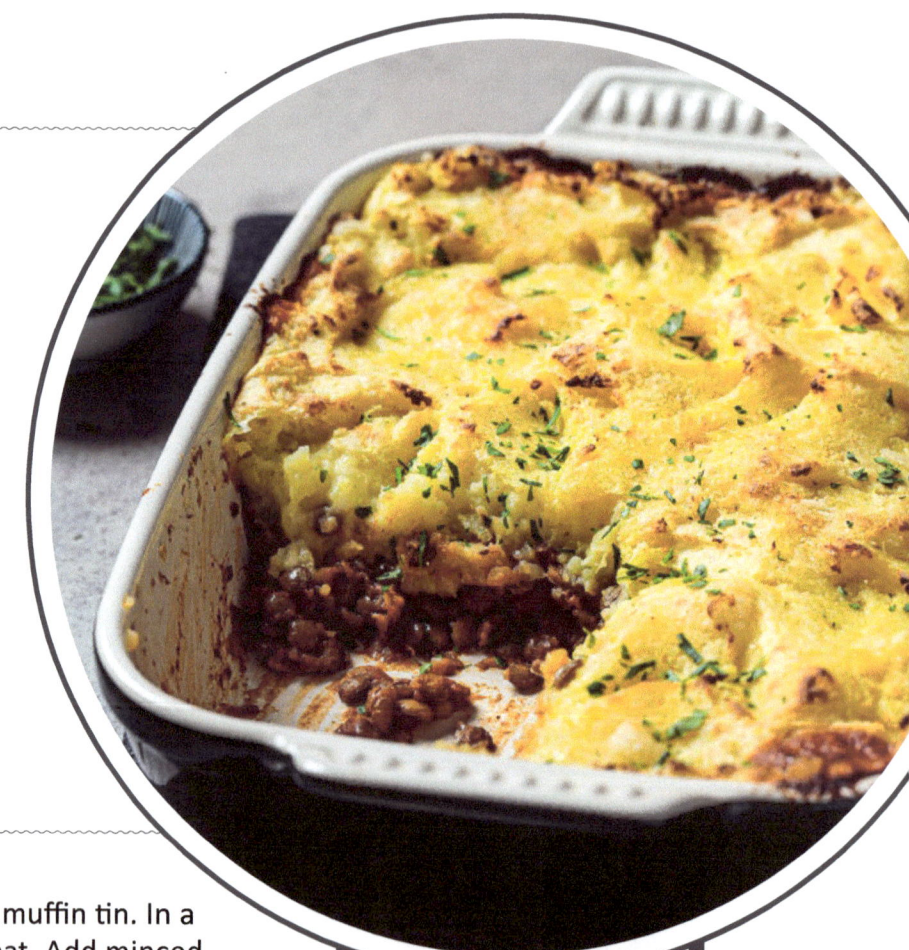

INSTRUCTIONS

1. Preheat oven to 375°F (190°C). Grease a muffin tin. In a skillet, heat one tbsp oil over medium heat. Add minced beef and cook until browned. Drain any excess fat.
2. Add mixed vegetables, beef broth, tomato paste, stir properly. Cook for 5 minutes more until the mixture thickens. Powder it with salt and crushed pepper.
3. Spoon the beef mixture into the muffin tin cups and top with mashed potatoes.
4. Bake for 16-20 minutes. Let cool slightly before serving.

PREP TIME:
10 MINS

COOK TIME:
15 MINS

SERVING
4

NUTRITIONAL VALUES (PER SERVING)

Calories: 350, Protein: 20g, Carbohydrates: 35g, Fat: 15g, Fiber: 4g

SIMPLE CHICKEN ALFREDO

INGREDIENTS

8 oz fettuccine pasta
1 lb chicken breast, sliced into strips
1 cup heavy cream
1/2 cup grated Parmesan cheese
2 tablespoons butter
2 cloves garlic, minced
Salt and pepper to taste

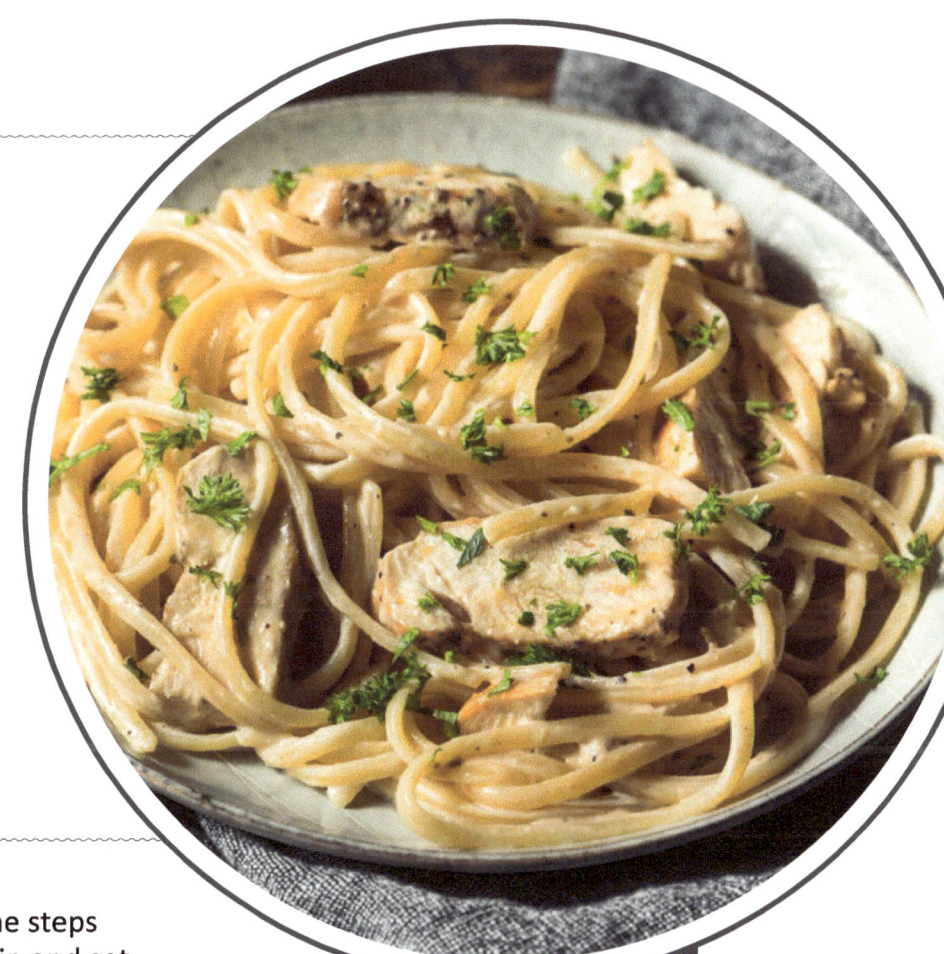

INSTRUCTIONS

1. Cook the fettuccine pasta according to the steps mentioned on the packet guidelines. Drain and set aside.
2. In a skillet, melt the butter. Add chicken strips and cook until fully cooked and browned, about 7-8 minutes. Remove chicken from skillet and set aside.
3. Use the same skillet, Add mashed garlic, and cook for 1 minute until fragrant.
4. Ladle in the heavy cream and bring to a simmer. Toss in the grated Parmesan cheese until the sauce is smooth and thickened.
5. Return the cooked chicken to the skillet and toss to coat with the Alfredo sauce. Serve over the cooked fettuccine pasta.

PREP TIME:
10 MINS

COOK TIME:
15 MINS

SERVING
4

NUTRITIONAL VALUES (PER SERVING)

Calories: 450, Protein: 30g, Carbohydrates: 35g, Fat: 20g, Fiber: 2g

Spaghetti Carbonara

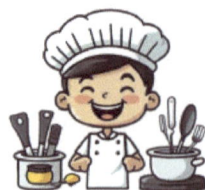

Ingredients

8 oz spaghetti

4 slices bacon, diced

2 large eggs

1/2 cup grated Parmesan cheese

2 cloves garlic, minced

Salt and pepper to taste

Fresh parsley, chopped (optional)

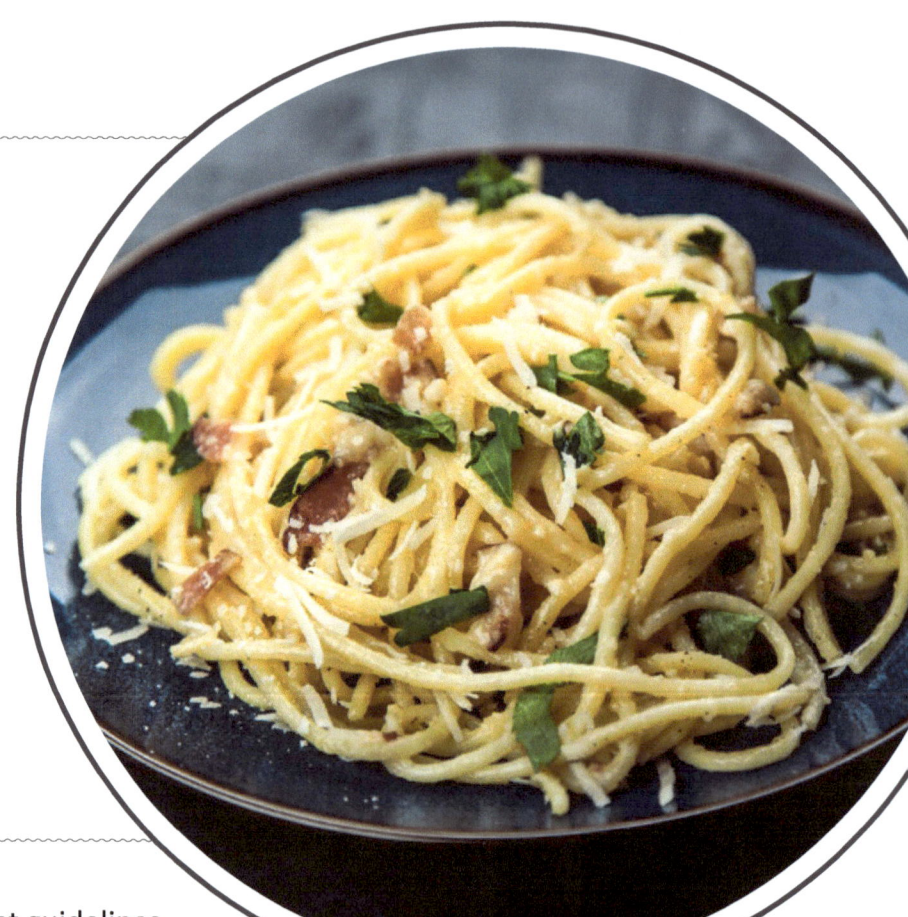

Instructions

1. Cook the spaghetti according to the packet guidelines. Reserve ½ cup of pasta water, drain the rest of the water, save the spaghetti for later, and set aside.
2. In a skillet, cook diced bacon until crispy. Remove the bacon pieces and set aside, leaving the bacon fat in the skillet.
3. Add mashed garlic to the skillet and cook for 1 minute until fragrant.
4. In a deep-bottom bowl, pulse the eggs and grated Parmesan cheese.
5. Add prepared spaghetti to the skillet with the garlic. Remove the skillet from heat and quickly pour the egg-cheese mixture over the pasta, tossing to coat. Add reserved water (use as needed) to achieve a creamy consistency.
6. Stir in the crispy bacon and Powder it with salt and crushed pepper. If desired, garnish with chopped parsley.

Nutritional Values (per serving)

Calories: 400, Protein: 18g, Carbohydrates: 45g, Fat: 15g, Fiber: 2g

PREP TIME:
10 MINS

COOK TIME:
15 MINS

SERVING
4

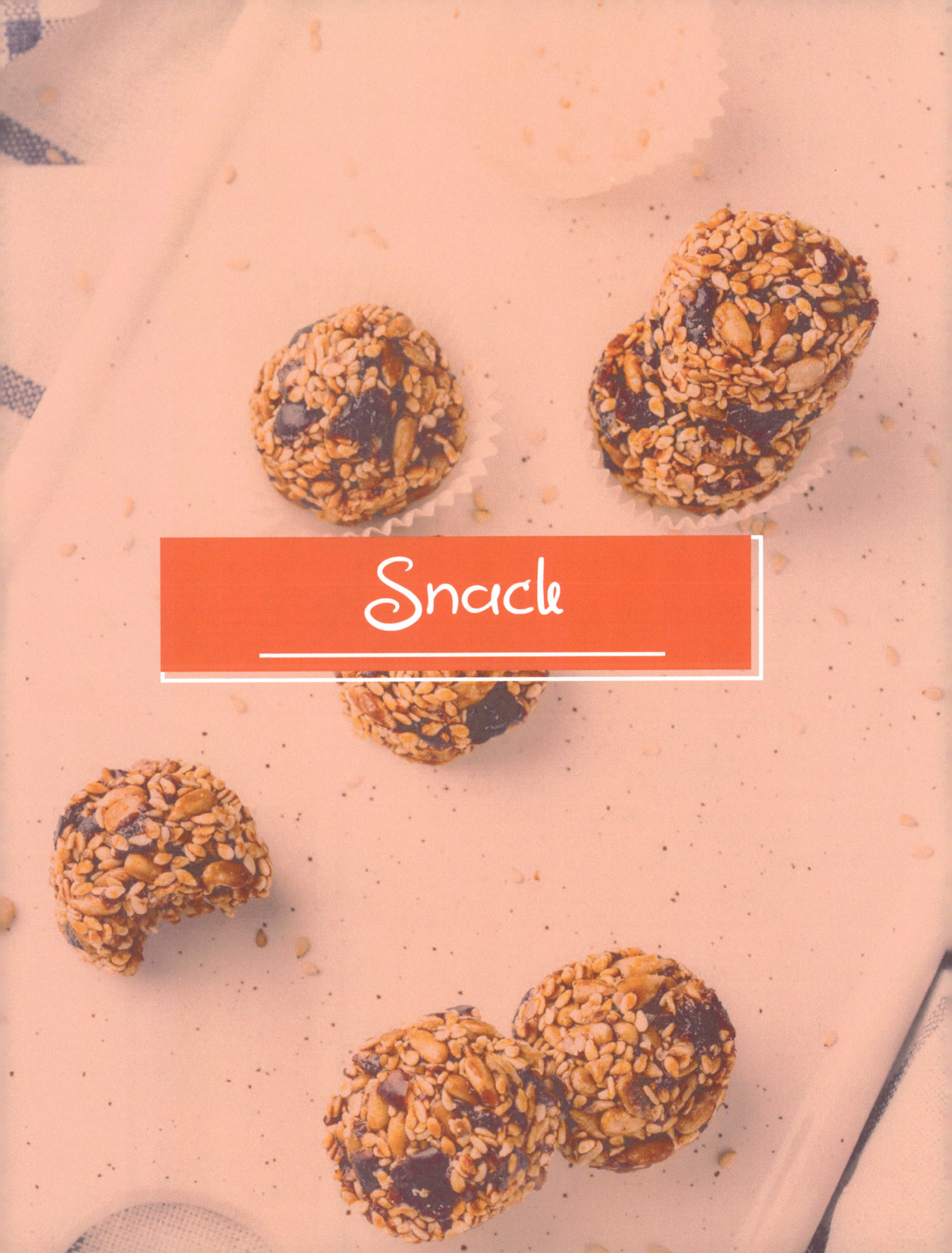

Snack

Veggie Sticks with Hummus

Ingredients

1 cup carrot sticks
1 cup cucumber sticks
1 cup bell pepper sticks
1 cup celery sticks
1 cup hummus

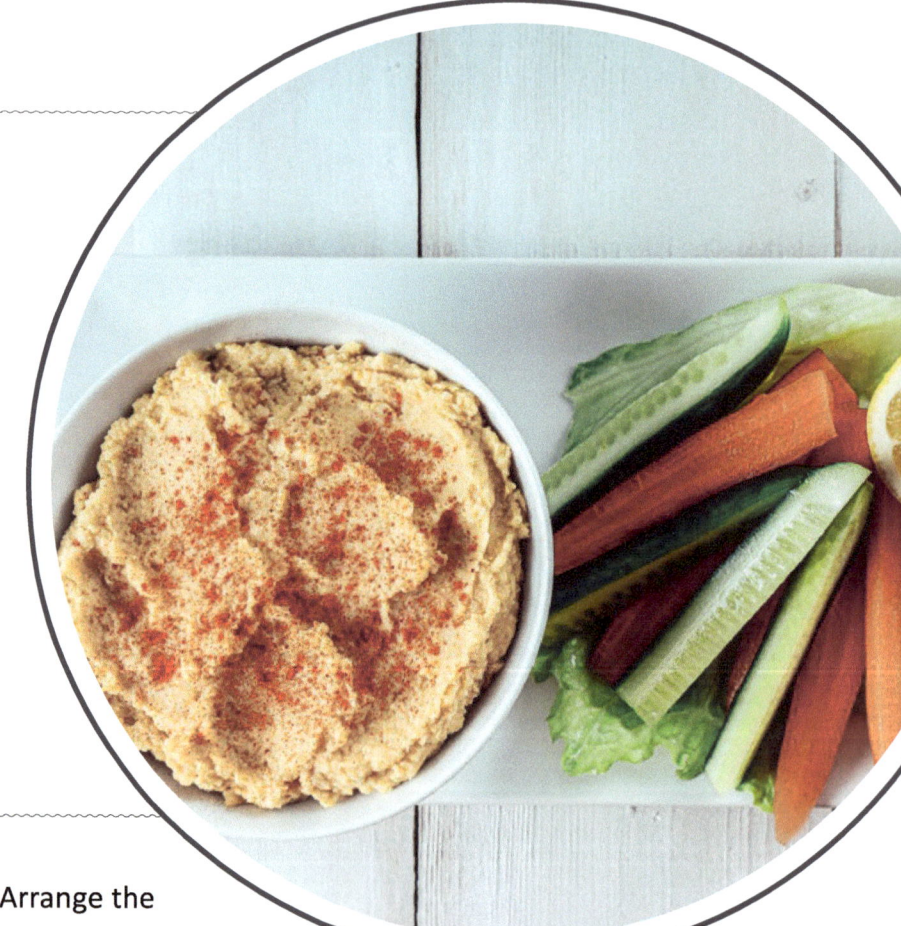

Instructions

1. Wash and cut the vegetables into sticks. Arrange the veggie sticks on a platter.
2. Place the hummus In a deep-bottom bowl in the center of the platter. Serve immediately, and enjoy dipping the veggie sticks in the hummus.

PREP TIME:
10 MINS

COOK TIME:
0 MINS

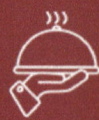

SERVING
4

Nutritional Values (per serving)

Calories: 120, Protein: 4g, Carbohydrates: 15g, Fat: 6g, Fiber: 5g

Apple Slices with Peanut Butter

Ingredients

2 apples, cored and sliced
1/4 cup peanut butter

Instructions

1. Wash the apples thoroughly. Core and slice the apples.
2. Arrange the apple slices on a plate. Serve with peanut butter as a side for dipping.

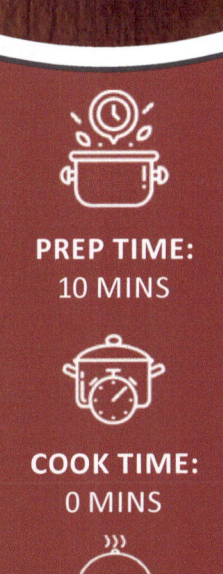

PREP TIME:
10 MINS

COOK TIME:
0 MINS

SERVING
4

Nutritional Values (per serving)

Calories: 180, Protein: 4g, Carbohydrates: 28g, Fat: 8g, Fiber: 5g

Cheese and Crackers

Ingredients

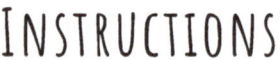

1/4 lb cheese from a cheese
block (cheddar, mozzarella, or
your favorite cheese)
12 whole grain crackers
1 apple or pear
Jam or jelly or peanut butter
(you choose!)
1/4 cup of chopped nuts (like
pecans, almonds or walnuts)
(optional)

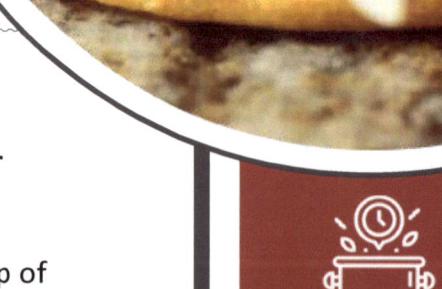

Instructions

1. Cut the cheese into small squares if not pre-cut.
   Arrange the cheese squares and crackers on a plate.
2. Cut apple or pear into small sections to fit on the
   cracker.
3. Add a small dab of jam, jelly or peanut butter on top of
   the cheese to each cracker.
4. Optional: Sprinkle nuts over the jam/jelly/peanut
   butter
5. Serve immediately and enjoy.

PREP TIME:
10 MINS

COOK TIME:
0 MINS

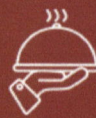

SERVING
2

Nutritional Values (per serving)

Calories: 200, Protein: 8g, Carbohydrates: 18g, Fat: 12g, Fiber: 2g

Ants on a Log

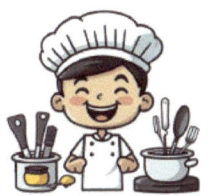

Ingredients

2 celery stalks, cut into 3-inch pieces
1/4 cup peanut butter
1/4 cup raisins

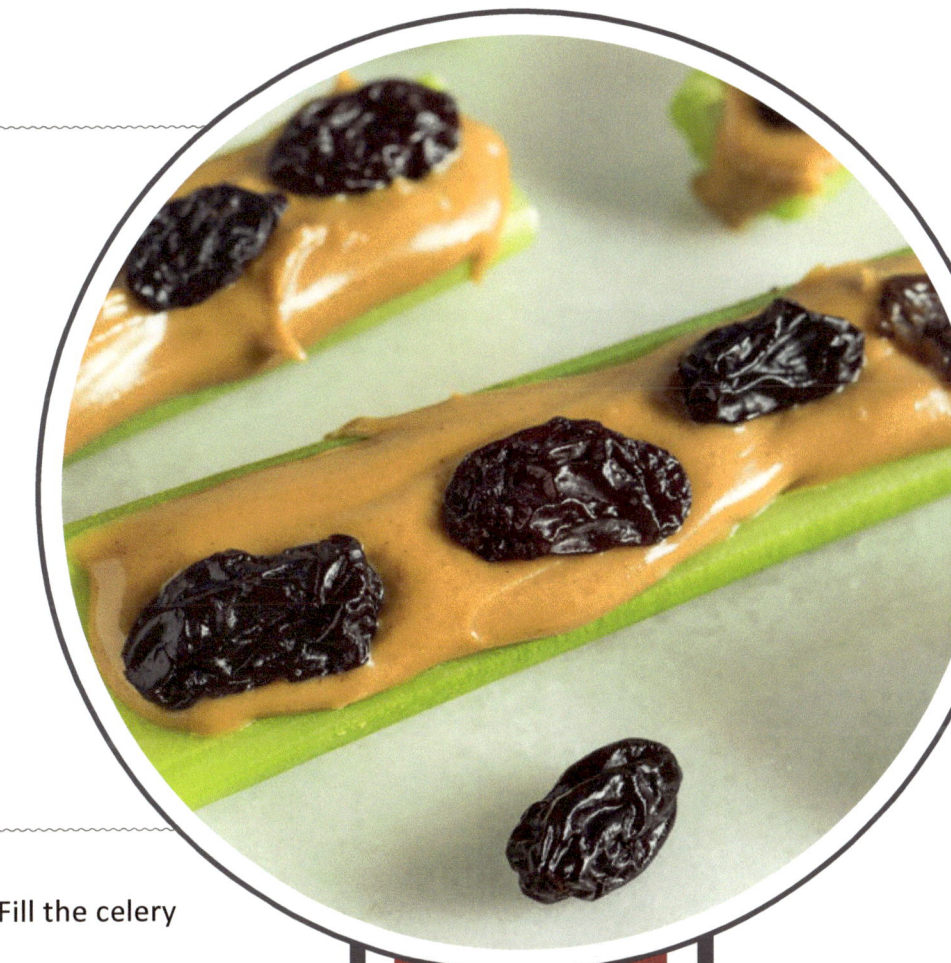

Instructions

1. Cut the celery stalks into 3-inch pieces. Fill the celery pieces with peanut butter.
2. Top with raisins to resemble ants on a log. Serve immediately and enjoy.

PREP TIME:
10 MINS

COOK TIME:
0 MINS

SERVING
2

Nutritional Values (per serving)

Calories: 150, Protein: 4g, Carbohydrates: 18g, Fat: 8g, Fiber: 3g

Fruit Kabobs

Ingredients

1 cup strawberries, hulled
1 cup pineapple chunks
1 cup grapes
1 cup melon balls
1 cup blueberries

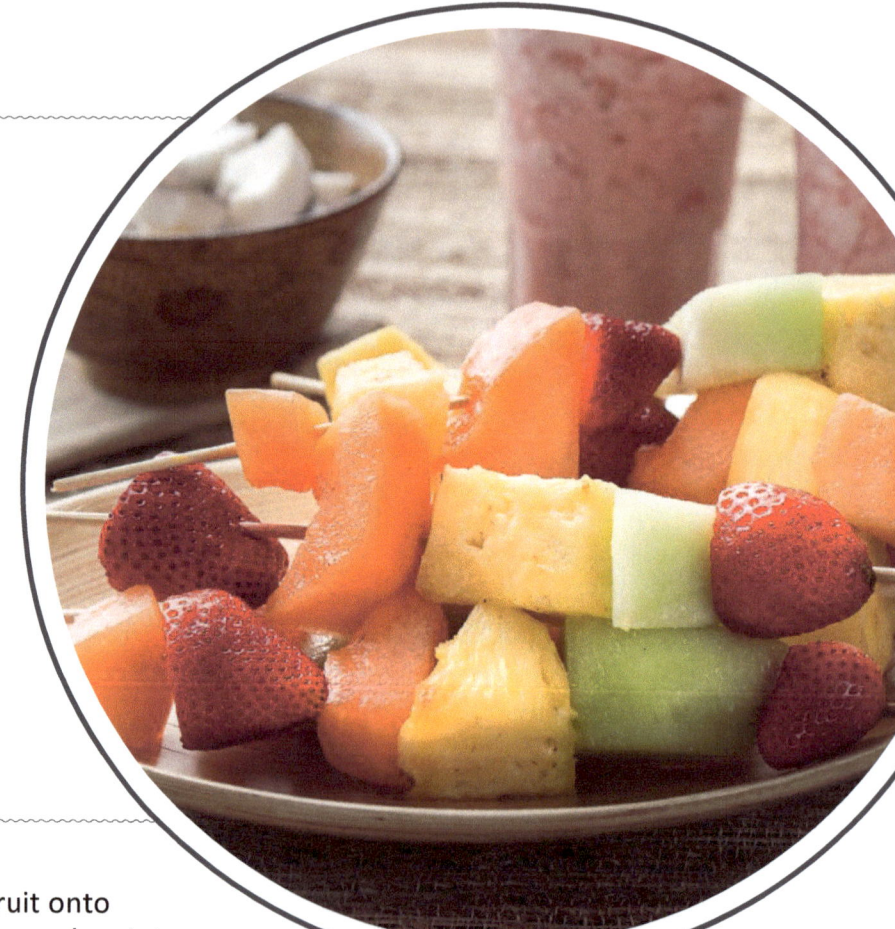

Instructions

1. Wash and prepare the fruit. Thread the fruit onto skewers, alternating types of fruit for color and variety.
2. Arrange the fruit kabobs on a platter and serve immediately.

PREP TIME:
10 MINS

COOK TIME:
0 MINS

SERVING
2

Nutritional Values (per serving)

Calories: 90, Protein: 1g, Carbohydrates: 22g, Fat: 0g, Fiber: 3g

Yogurt-Dipped Berries

Ingredients

1 cup strawberries
1 cup blueberries
1 cup Greek yogurt
1 tablespoon honey (optional)

Instructions

1. Wash the strawberries and blueberries. Dip the berries into the Greek yogurt, coating them evenly.
2. Arrange the yogurt-dipped berries on a plate. Drizzle honey, if desired, more sweetener, and serve immediately.

PREP TIME:
10 MINS

COOK TIME:
0 MINS

SERVING
2

Nutritional Values (per serving)

Calories: 100, Protein: 4g, Carbohydrates: 18g, Fat: 2g, Fiber: 3g

Trail Mix

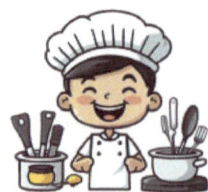

Ingredients

1/2 cup almonds
1/2 cup raisins
1/2 cup sunflower seeds
1/2 cup chocolate chips
1/2 cup dried cranberries

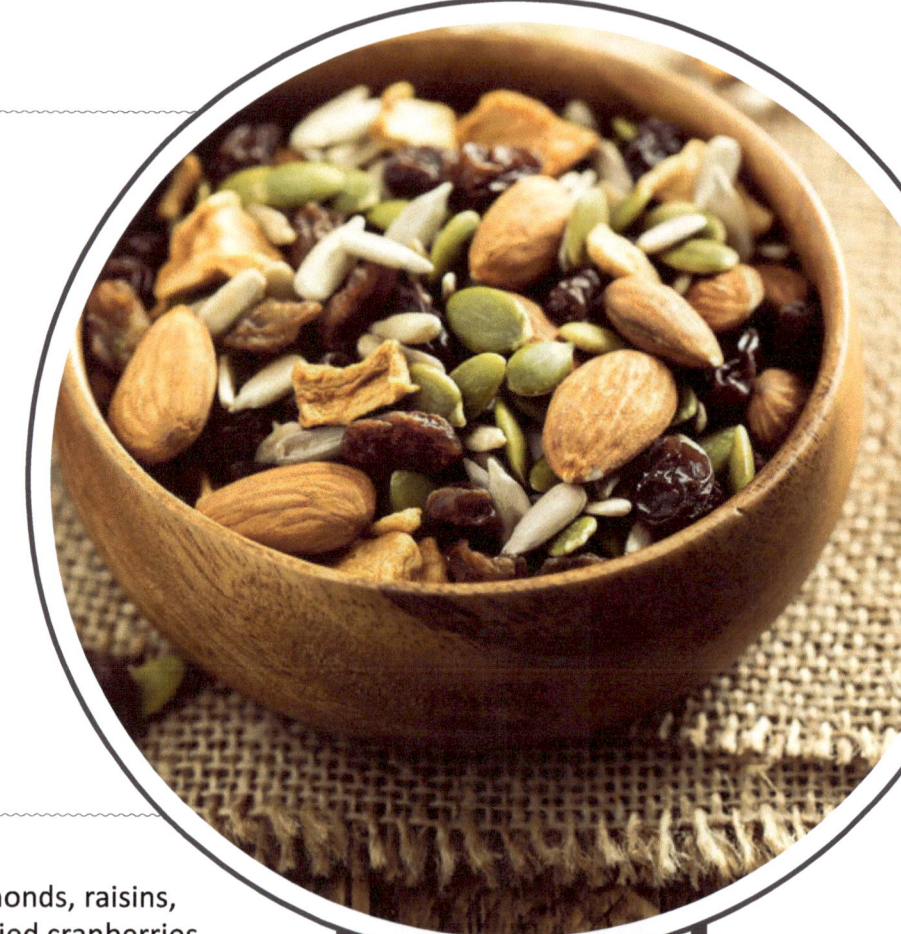

Instructions

1. In a deep-bottom bowl, combine the almonds, raisins, sunflower seeds, chocolate chips, and dried cranberries.
2. Mix well to combine. Divide into portions and serve.

PREP TIME:
10 MINS

COOK TIME:
0 MINS

SERVING
4

Nutritional Values (per serving)

Calories: 200, Protein: 4g, Carbohydrates: 28g, Fat: 10g, Fiber: 3g

Cucumber Sandwiches

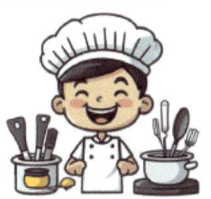

Ingredients

1 cucumber, sliced thin
8 slices whole grain bread
1/4 cup cream cheese
1 tablespoon fresh dill, chopped
Salt and pepper to taste

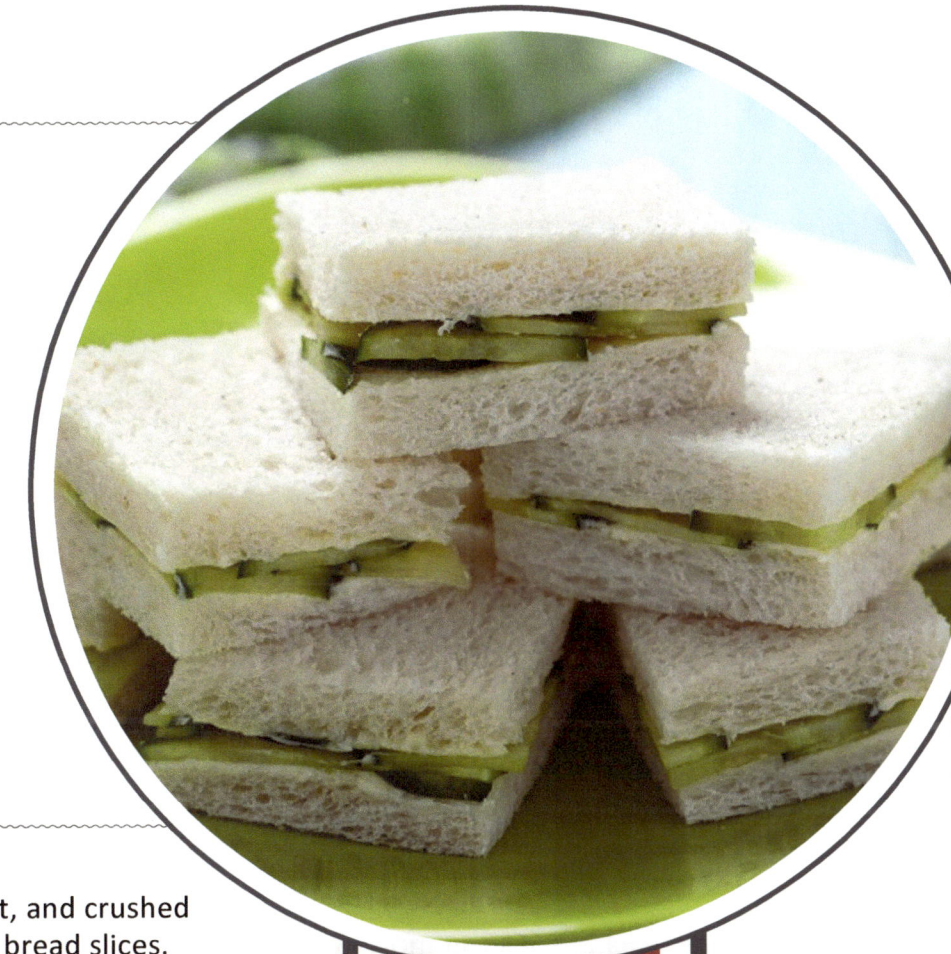

Instructions

1. Mix the cream cheese with fresh dill, salt, and crushed pepper. Spread the cheese mixture over bread slices.
2. Arrange cucumber slices on top of the four slices of bread. Top with slices of leftover bread to make sandwiches.
3. Cut the sandwiches into pieces (quarters) and serve immediately.

PREP TIME:
10 MINS

COOK TIME:
0 MINS

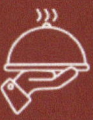

SERVING
4

Nutritional Values (per serving)

Calories: 150, Protein: 4g, Carbohydrates: 22g, Fat: 6g, Fiber: 3g

Banana Sushi

Ingredients

2 bananas
1/4 cup peanut butter
1/4 cup granola
1 tablespoon honey (optional)

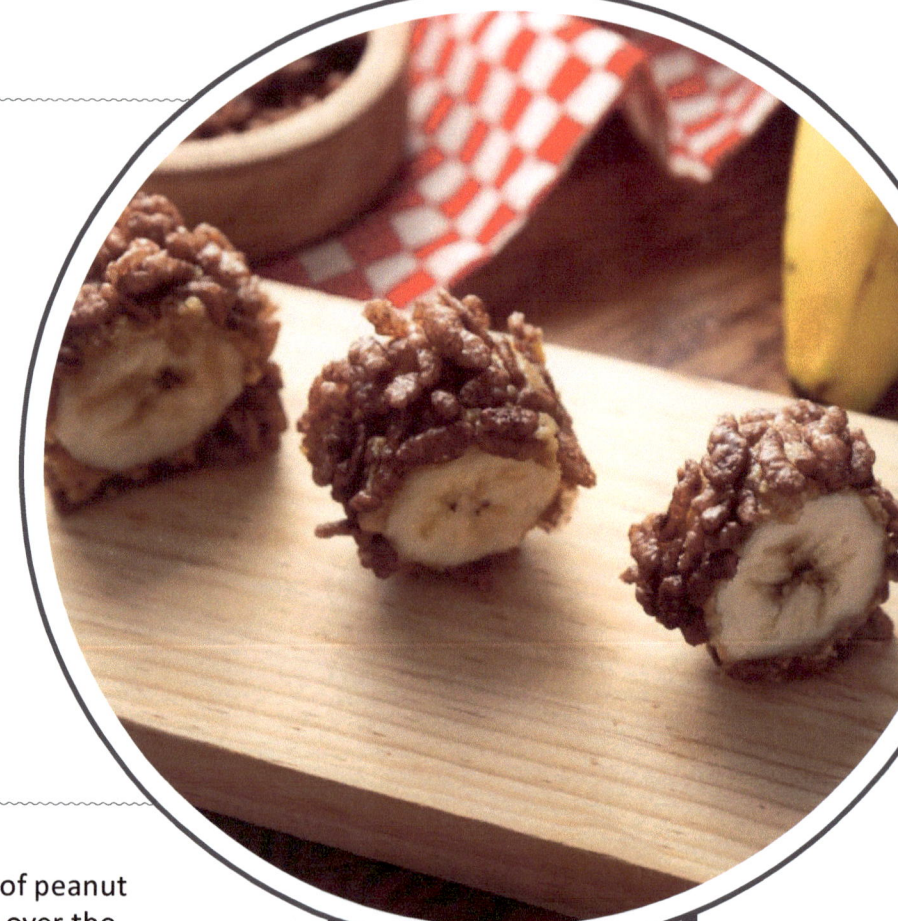

Instructions

1. Peel the bananas and spread a thin layer of peanut butter over each. Sprinkle granola evenly over the peanut butter.
2. Drizzle with honey if desired. Slice the bananas into bite-sized pieces and serve immediately.

PREP TIME:
10 MINS

COOK TIME:
0 MINS

SERVING
4

Nutritional Values (per serving)

Calories: 200, Protein: 5g, Carbohydrates: 35g, Fat: 8g, Fiber: 4g

Cinnamon Apple Chips

Ingredients

2 large apples, cored and thinly sliced
1 teaspoon cinnamon
1 tablespoon sugar (optional)

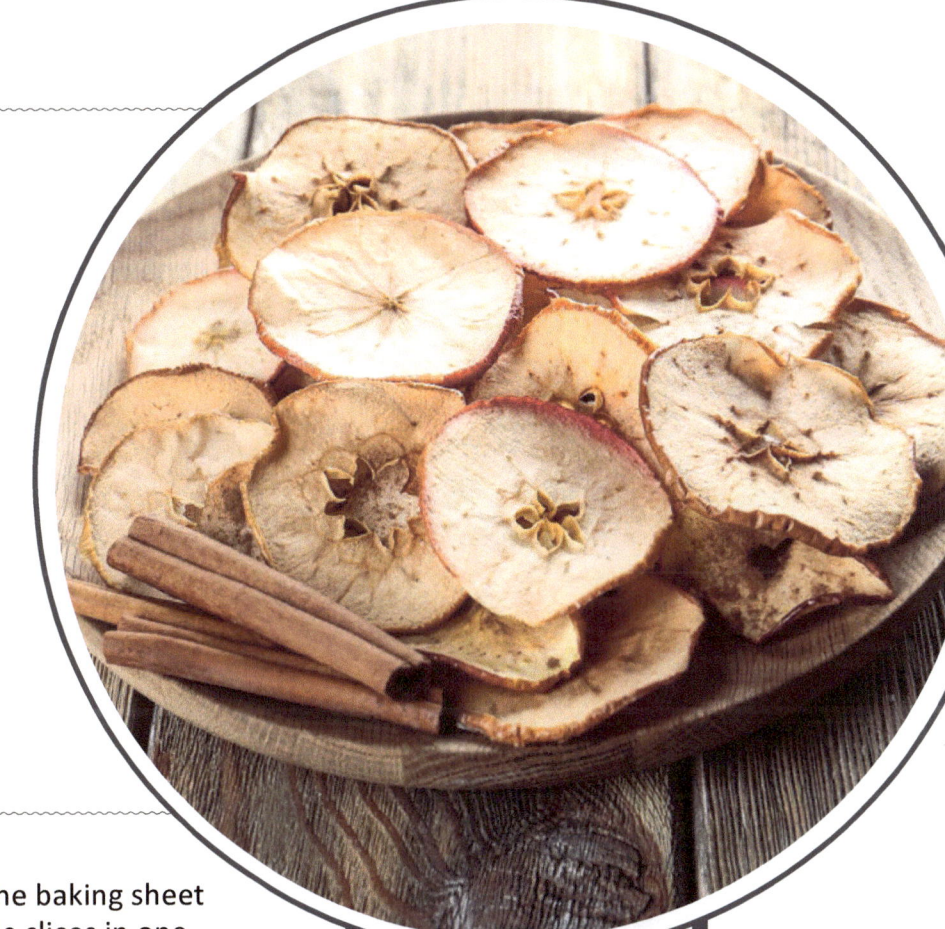

Instructions

1. Preheat oven to 200°F (95°C). Arrange the baking sheet with parchment paper. Arrange the apple slices in one layer on the baking sheet.
2. In a deep-bottom bowl, mix the cinnamon and sugar (if using). Sprinkle the cinnamon mixture evenly over the apple slices.
3. Bake for 2 hours until the apple slices are crisp, turning them halfway through the baking time.
4. Let the apple chips cool completely before serving.

PREP TIME:
10 MINS

COOK TIME:
5 MINS

SERVING
4

Nutritional Values (per serving)

Calories: 50, Protein: 0g, Carbohydrates: 14g, Fat: 0g, Fiber: 3g

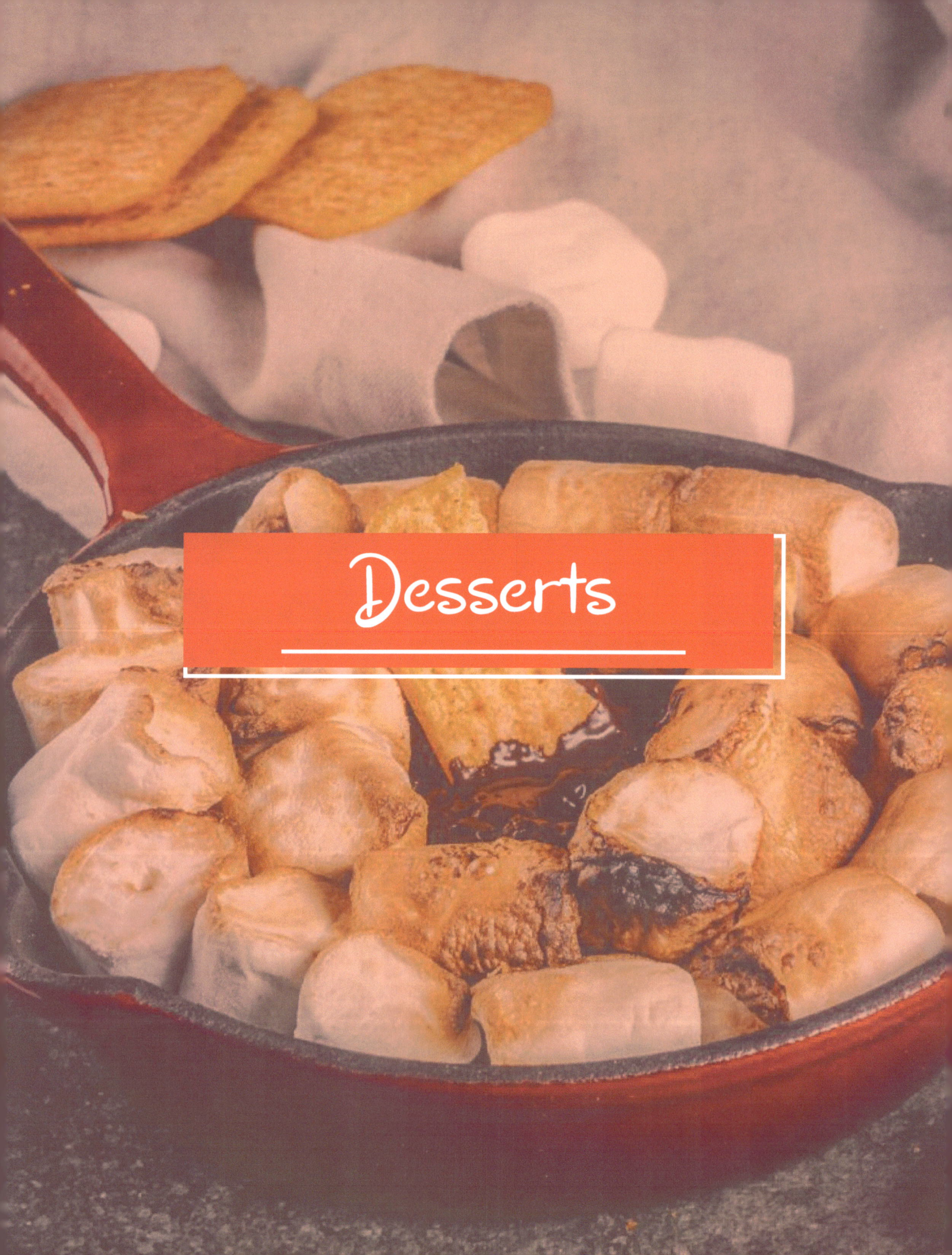

Desserts

Fruit Parfait

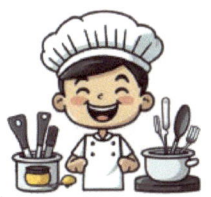

Ingredients

1 cup Greek yogurt
1 cup mixed berries (strawberries, blueberries, raspberries)
1/2 cup granola
1 tablespoon honey (optional)

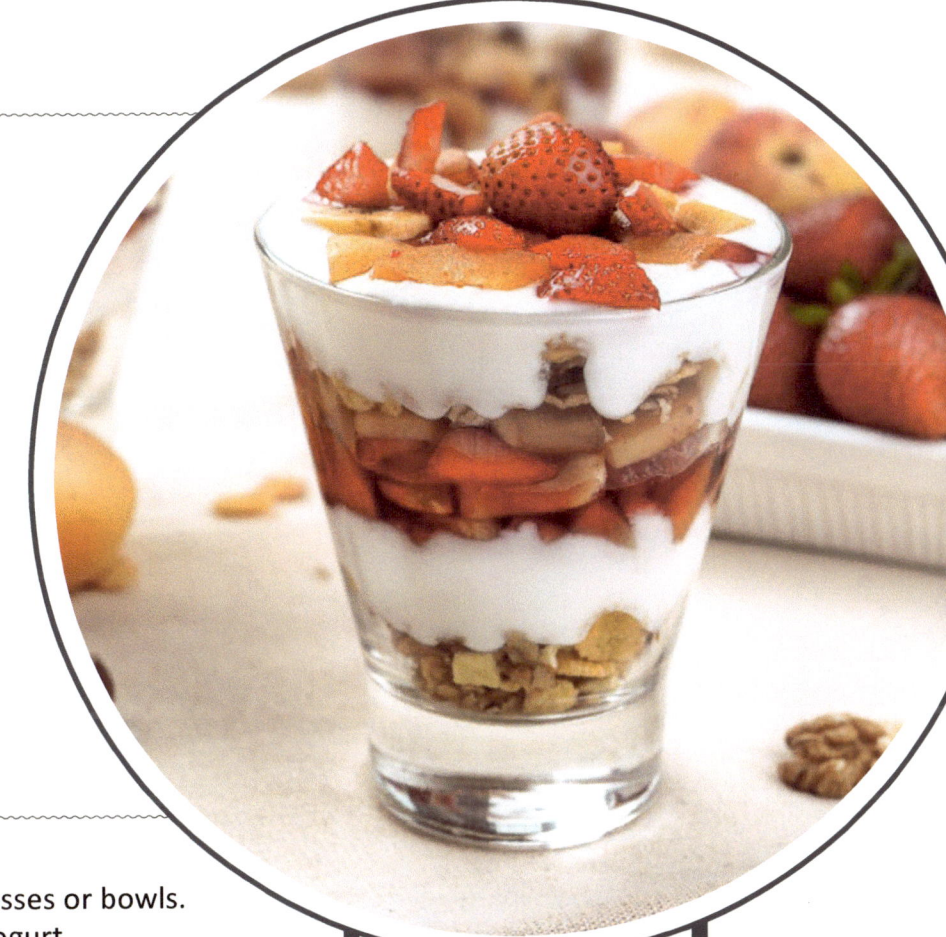

Instructions

1. Layer half of the Greek yogurt in two glasses or bowls. Place the mixed berries layer over the yogurt.
2. Sprinkle granola over the berries. Repeat the layers with the leftover yogurt, berries, and granola.
3. Drizzle honey, if desired, more sweetener, and serve immediately.

PREP TIME:
10 MINS

COOK TIME:
0 MINS

SERVING
2

Nutritional Values (per serving)

Calories: 200, Protein: 10g, Carbohydrates: 30g, Fat: 5g, Fiber: 4g

CHOCOLATE DIPPED PRETZELS

INGREDIENTS

1 cup pretzel rods or mini pretzels
1/2 cup chocolate chips
1 tablespoon sprinkles (optional)

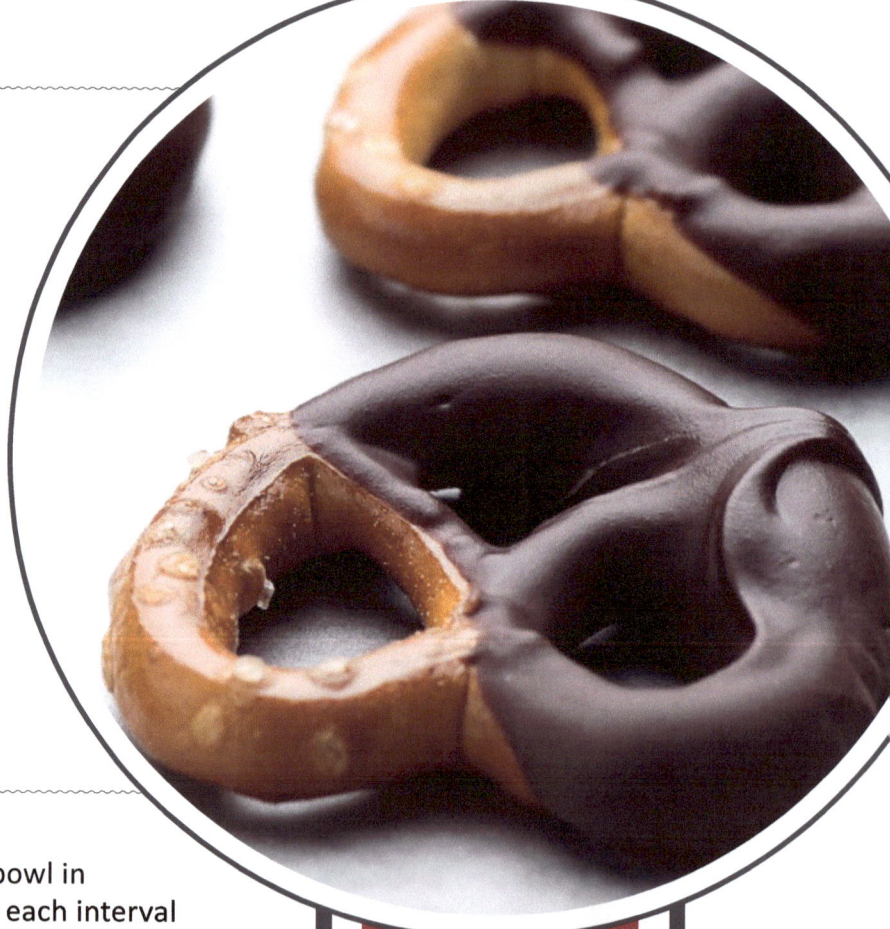

INSTRUCTIONS

1. Melt the chocolate chips in a heavy glass bowl in 30-second intervals and stir properly after each interval until smooth.
2. Dip each pretzel rod or mini pretzel halfway into the melted chocolate. Place the chocolate-dipped pretzels on a sheet of parchment paper.
3. Sprinkle with sprinkles if desired. Allow the chocolate to set before serving.

PREP TIME:
10 MINS

COOK TIME:
5 MINS

SERVING
4

NUTRITIONAL VALUES (PER SERVING)

Calories: 150, Protein: 2g, Carbohydrates: 25g, Fat: 6g, Fiber: 1g

Fruit Popsicles

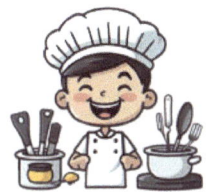

Ingredients

2 cups mixed fruit (mango, strawberries, blueberries, kiwi)
1 cup fruit juice (orange, apple, or
your choice)
1 tablespoon honey (optional)

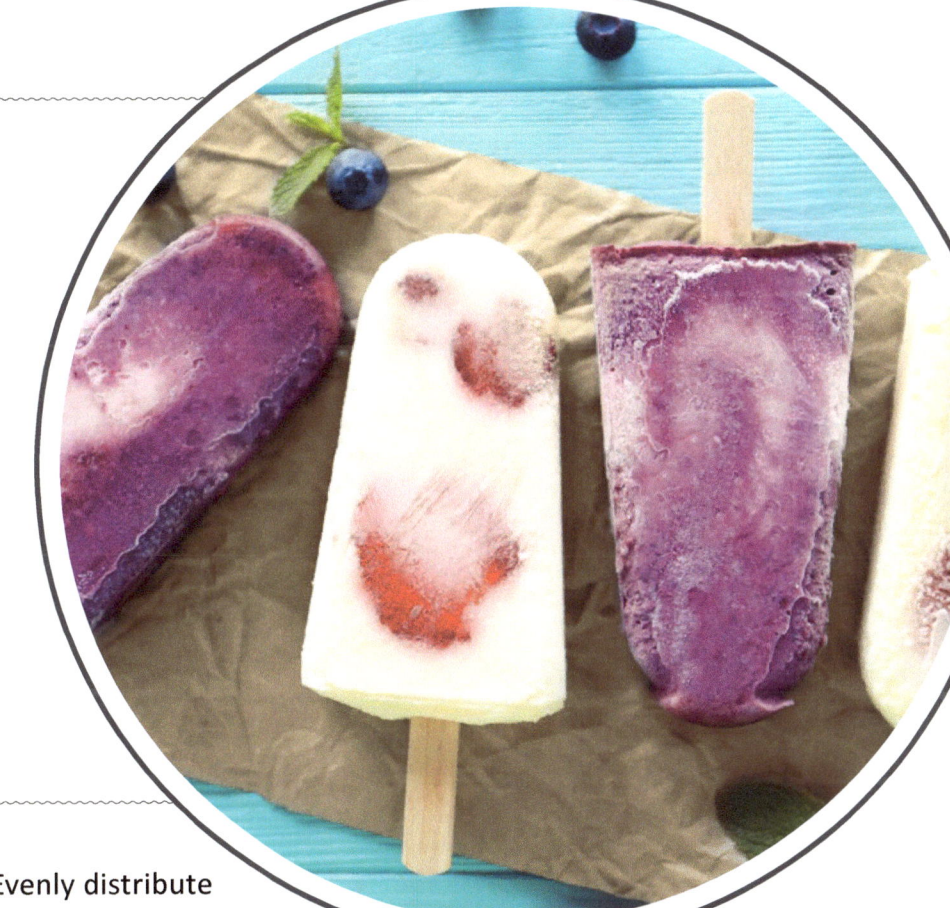

Instructions

1. Chop the mixed fruit into small pieces. Evenly distribute the fruit pieces into popsicle molds.
2. Pour the fruit juice over the fruit in the molds. Add honey to the juice if desired for extra sweetness.
3. Insert popsicle sticks and leave to freeze for 4 hours (at least) or until completely frozen. Remove the popsicles and serve.

PREP TIME:
10 MINS

COOK TIME:
0 MINS

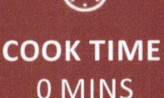

SERVING
2

Nutritional Values (per serving)

Calories: 80, Protein: 1g, Carbohydrates: 20g, Fat: 0g, Fiber: 2g

Rice Krispie Treats

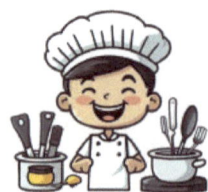

Ingredients

3 cups Rice Krispies cereal
2 tablespoons butter
2 cups mini marshmallows

Instructions

1. In a pot, melt the butter. Add mini marshmallows and stir to ensure they are completely melted.
2. Remove and stir in the Rice Krispies cereal properly until well coated. With the spatula, press the mixture into a greased 8x8-inch pan.
3. Cool and set before cutting and serving.

PREP TIME:
10 MINS

COOK TIME:
5 MINS

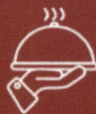

SERVING
4

Nutritional Values (per serving)

Calories: 150, Protein: 1g, Carbohydrates: 30g, Fat: 4g, Fiber: 0g

S'mores Dip

Ingredients

1 cup chocolate chips
1 cup mini marshmallows
1/2 cup crushed graham crackers
Graham crackers for dipping

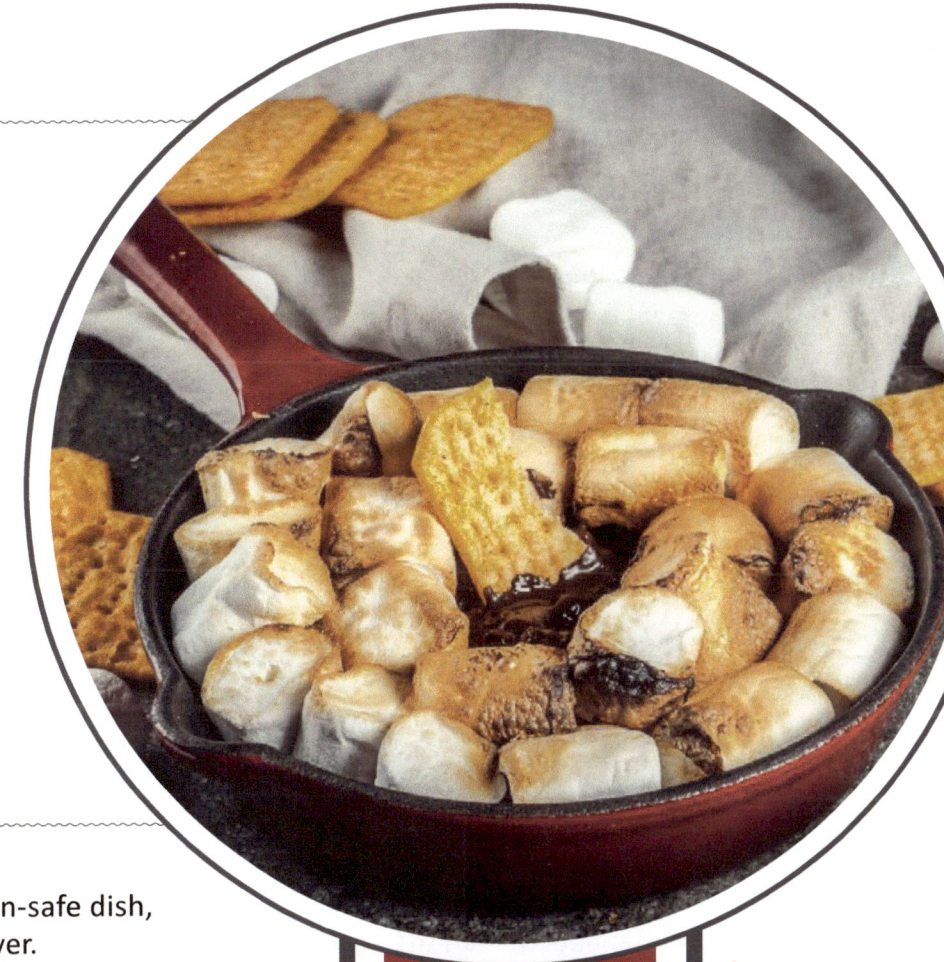

Instructions

1. Preheat oven to 350°F (175°C). In an oven-safe dish, spread the chocolate chips in an even layer.
2. Top with an even layer of mini marshmallows.
3. Bake for 4-5 minutes until golden brown and the chocolate is melted.
4. Sprinkle crushed graham crackers and serve immediately with graham crackers for dipping.

PREP TIME:
10 MINS

COOK TIME:
5 MINS

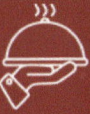

SERVING
2

Nutritional Values (per serving)

Calories: 200, Protein: 2g, Carbohydrates: 40g, Fat: 7g, Fiber: 1g

Frozen Yogurt Bark

Ingredients

2 cups Greek yogurt
1/4 cup honey
1/2 cup mixed berries (strawberries, blueberries, raspberries)
1/4 cup granola

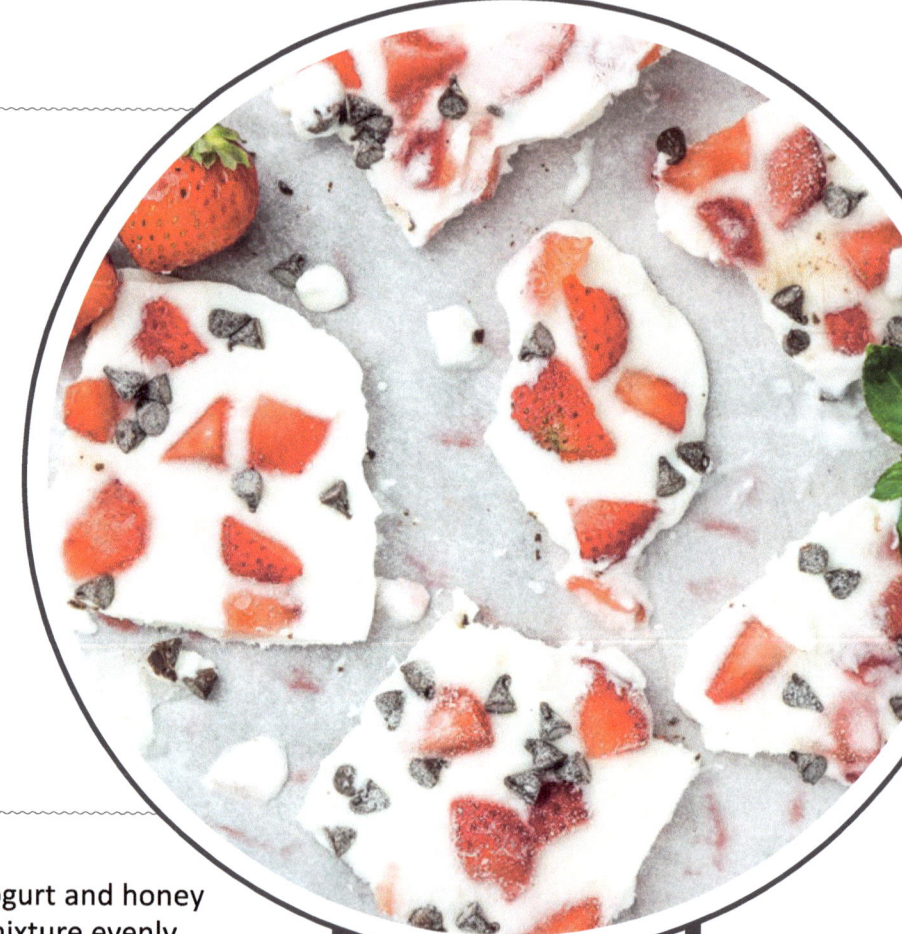

Instructions

1. In a deep-bottom bowl, mix the Greek yogurt and honey until well combined. Spread the yogurt mixture evenly on a parchment-lined baking sheet.
2. Sprinkle the mixed berries and granola over the yogurt. Freeze for at least 2 hours or until completely frozen.
3. Break into pieces and serve.

PREP TIME:
10 MINS

COOK TIME:
5 MINS

SERVING
4

Nutritional Values (per serving)

Calories: 120, Protein: 6g, Carbohydrates: 22g, Fat: 2g, Fiber: 2g

Banana Splits

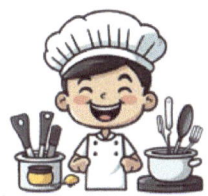

Ingredients

2 bananas, split lengthwise
1 cup vanilla ice cream
1/2 cup mixed berries (strawberries, blueberries, raspberries)
1/4 cup chocolate syrup
Whipped cream (optional)

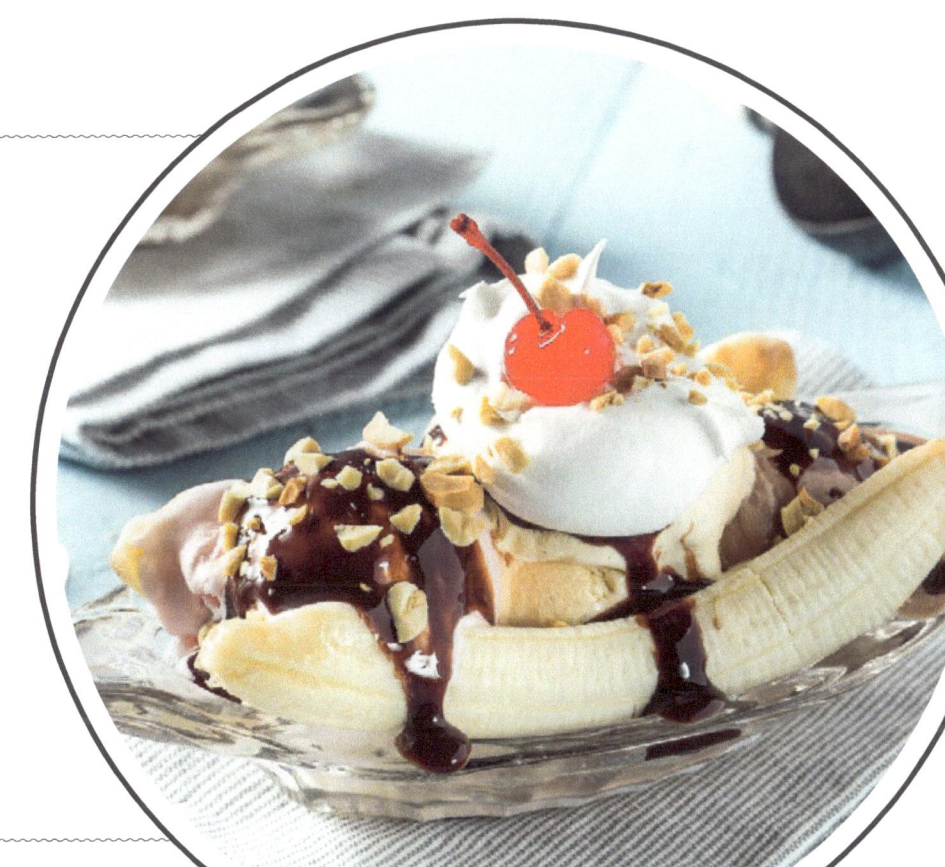

Instructions

1. Place the split bananas in the serving dishes. Add vanilla ice cream between the banana halves.
2. Top with mixed berries. Drizzle with chocolate syrup. Add whipped cream if desired to taste the creamy texture, and serve immediately.

PREP TIME:
10 MINS

COOK TIME:
5 MINS

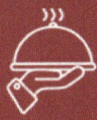

SERVING
2

Nutritional Values (per serving)

Calories: 250, Protein: 4g, Carbohydrates: 45g, Fat: 7g, Fiber: 4g

FRUIT SORBET

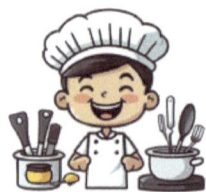

INGREDIENTS

2 cups frozen fruit (mango, strawberries, or your choice)
1/4 cup honey
1/2 cup water
1 tablespoon lemon juice

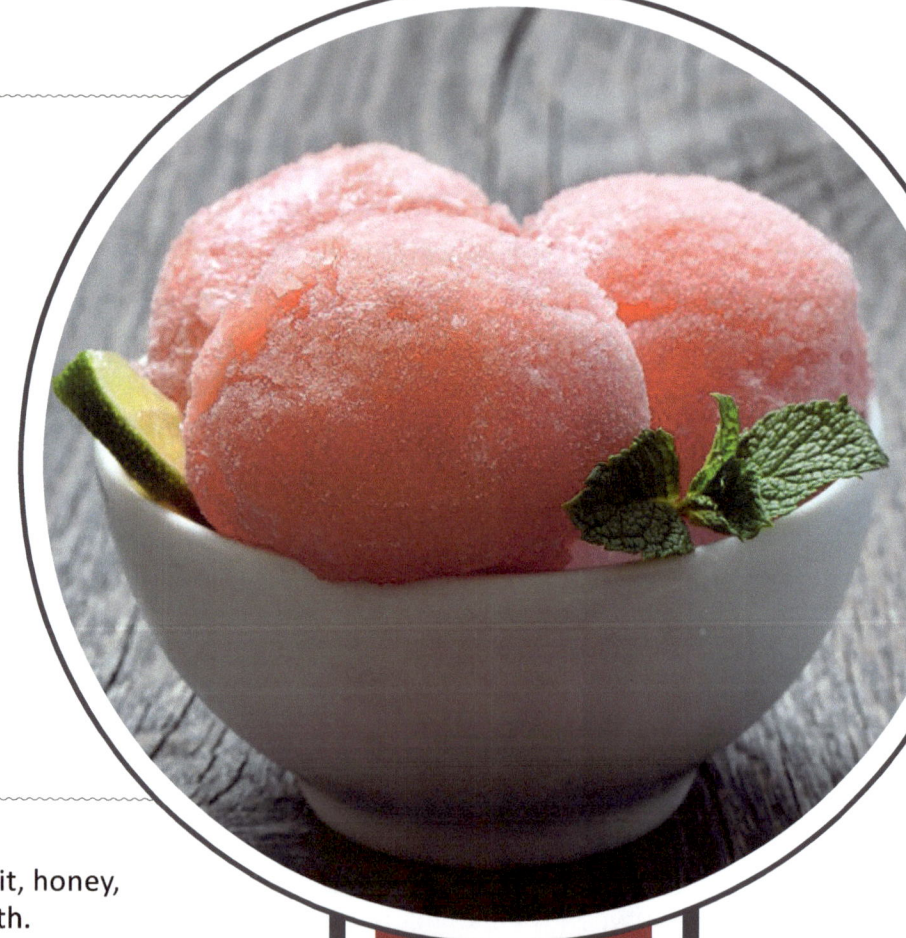

INSTRUCTIONS

1. In a food blender, combine the frozen fruit, honey,
    water, and lemon juice. Blend until smooth.
2. Pour the mixture into a deep-bottom container and freeze for 2
    hours to firm. Scoop into bowls and serve.

PREP TIME:
10 MINS

COOK TIME:
5 MINS

SERVING
4

NUTRITIONAL VALUES (PER SERVING)

Calories: 100, Protein: 1g, Carbohydrates: 26g, Fat: 0g, Fiber: 2g

Almond Stuffed Dates

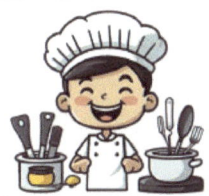

Ingredients

12 large dates, pitted
12 whole almonds
1/4 cup shredded coconut (optional)

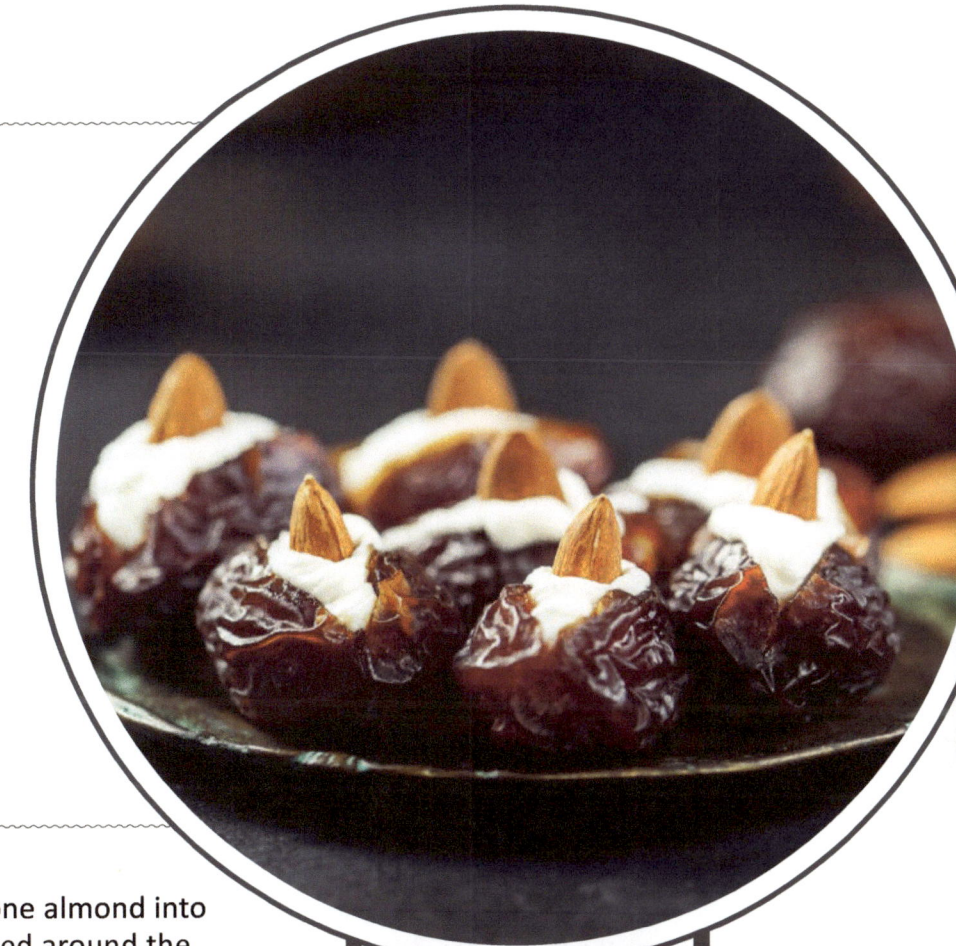

Instructions

1. Carefully open each pitted date. Insert one almond into each date and gently press the date closed around the almond.
2. Roll the stuffed dates in shredded coconut if desired. Arrange on a serving plate/dish and serve immediately.

PREP TIME:
10 MINS

COOK TIME:
5 MINS

SERVING
2

Nutritional Values (per serving)

Calories: 120, Protein: 2g, Carbohydrates: 24g, Fat: 3g, Fiber: 3g

Mug Brownie

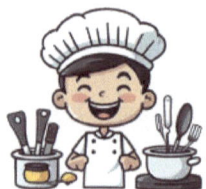

Ingredients

3 tablespoons flour
2 tablespoons of white sugar
1 tablespoon of cocoa powder
1/4 teaspoon of baking powder
1 tablespoon of vegetable oil
3 tablespoons of milk (or water)
2 tablespoons of chocolate chips
1/4 teaspoon of vanilla extract
Pinch of salt to taste

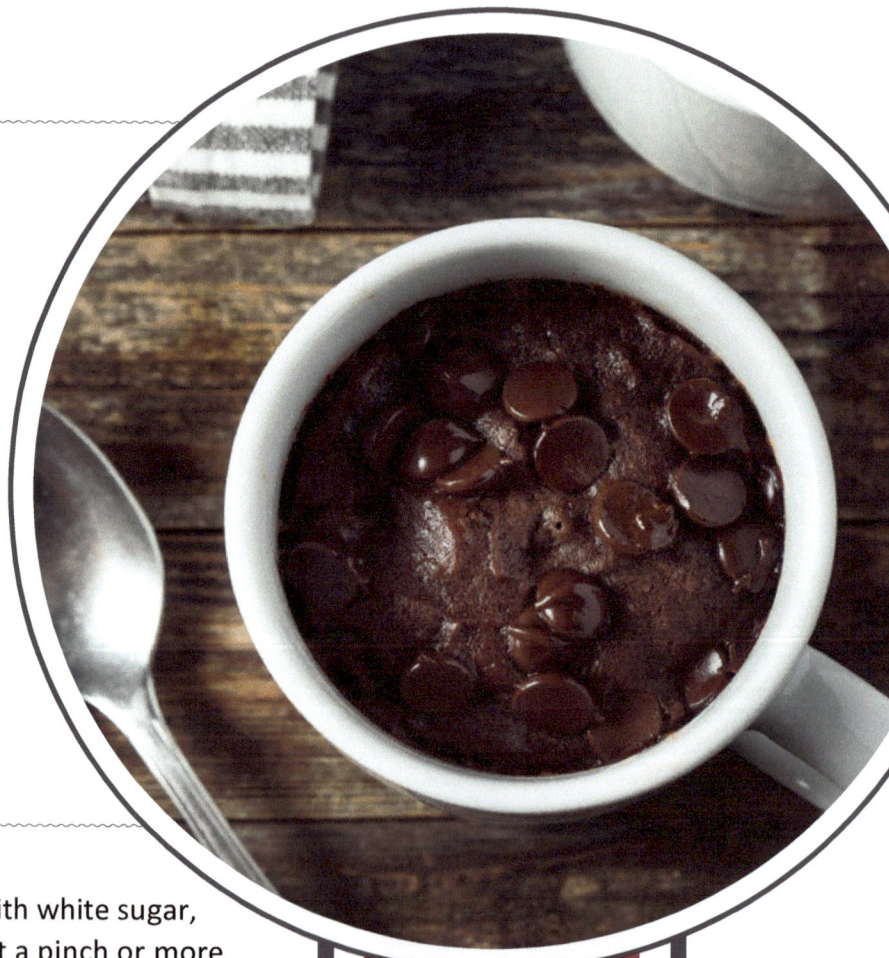

Instructions

1. Using a fork or small whisk, toss the flour with white sugar, baking powder, cocoa powder, and salt (just a pinch or more to taste) in a microwave-safe mug (12oz or 16 oz).

2. Add vegetable oil, milk and vanilla extract and stir until smooth. Stir in chocolate chips. Microwave on high for about 60-70 seconds until it is cooked through. May need an extra 10 seconds depending on mug size. Throw a few chocolate chips on top for the last 10 seconds if you want!

   Let cool slightly before enjoying directly from the mug.

   Great for sharing!

Nutritional Values (per serving)

Calories: 350, Protein: 2g, Carbohydrates: 60g, Fat: 15g, Fiber: 3g

PREP TIME:
10 MINS

COOK TIME:
5 MINS

SERVING
4

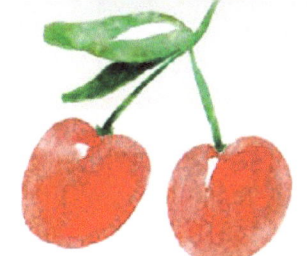
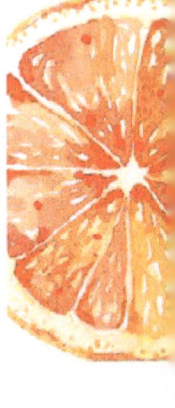

CONCLUSION

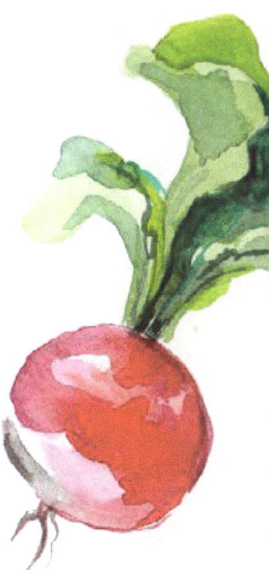

Congratulations, little chefs! You've reached the end of the "Hello Kids Cookbook." What an incredible journey it has been! From whipping up simple breakfasts to crafting delightful desserts, you've learned so much about the joy of cooking.

Cooking is more than just making food—it's about creativity, exploration, and sharing. By trying out these recipes, you've discovered new flavors, practiced important skills, and perhaps even found a new hobby that you love. Each dish you've made is a testament to your hard work and enthusiasm in the kitchen.

Remember, cooking is a skill that will serve you for a lifetime. Whether you're making a quick snack or preparing a meal for your family, the abilities you've gained from this cookbook will always come in handy. Don't be afraid to experiment with ingredients, try new recipes, and make each dish your own. The kitchen is your playground, and every recipe is a new adventure waiting to happen.

We hope this cookbook has inspired you to continue your culinary journey. Share your creations with family and friends, and enjoy the smiles and satisfaction that come from serving a meal made with love. Keep practicing, stay curious, and most importantly, have fun in the kitchen.

Thank you for joining us in this culinary adventure. We can't wait to see what you'll cook up next. Happy cooking, and remember to always greet each new recipe with a cheerful "Hello!"

Bon appétit!

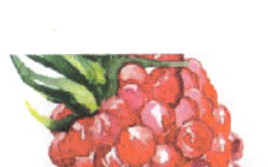

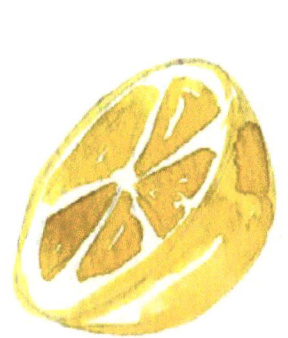

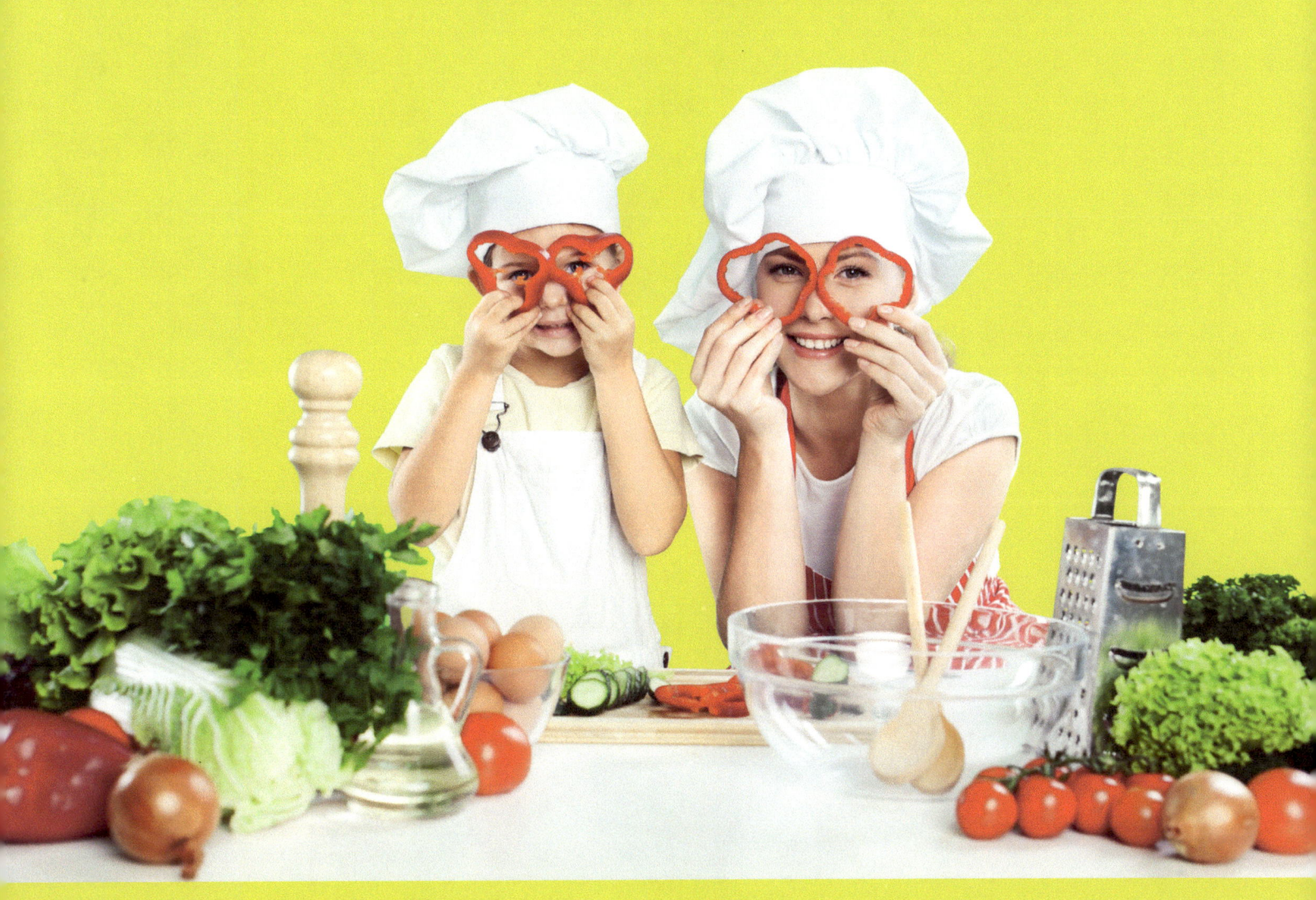

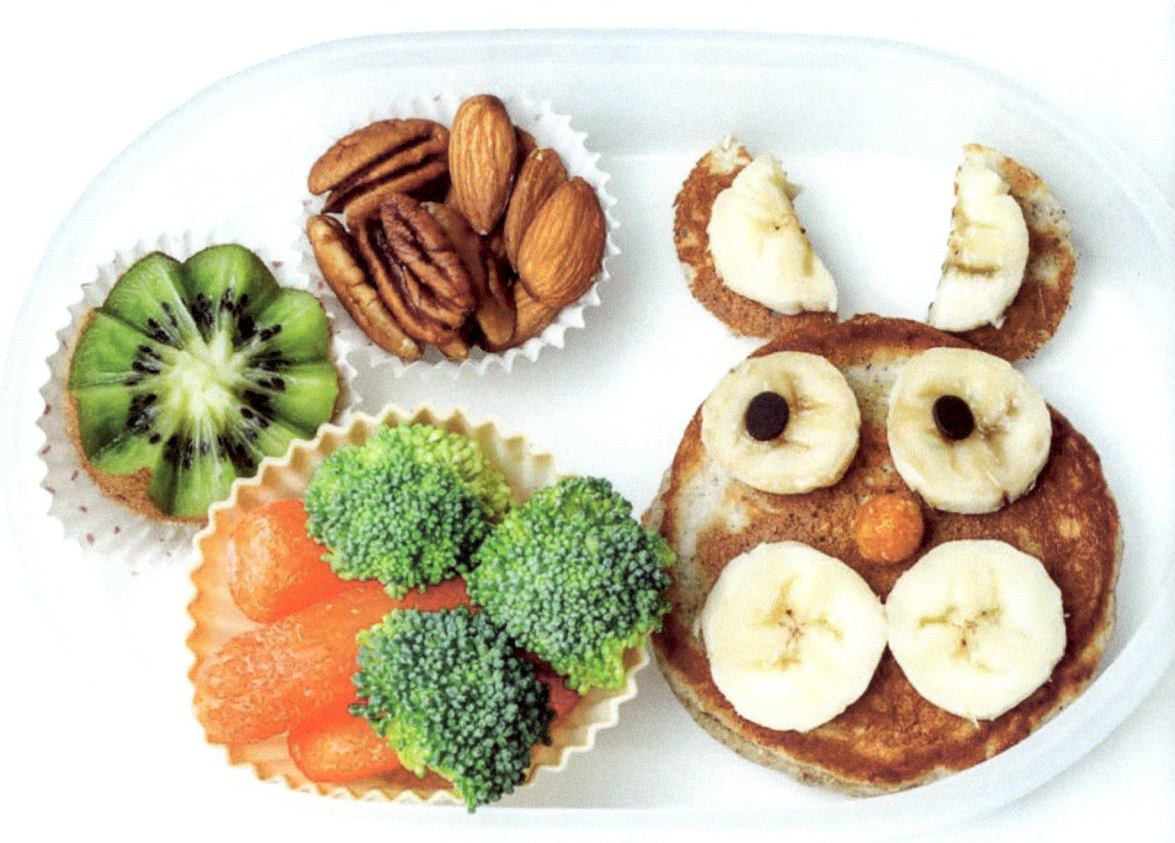
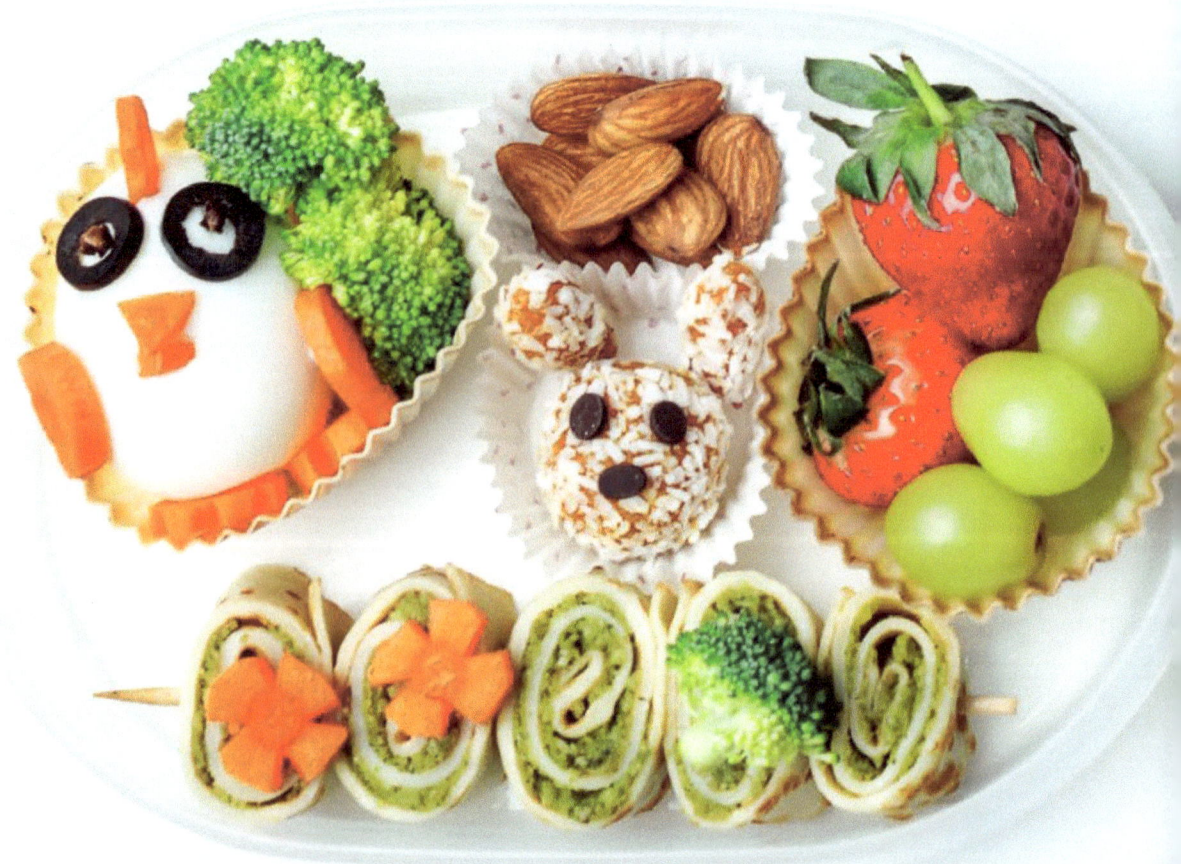